Particip
in Palliat

Participatory Research in Palliative Care
Actions and Reflections

Edited by

Jo Hockley
Nurse Consultant
St Christopher's Hospice
London, UK

Katherine Froggatt
Senior Lecturer
International Observatory on End of Life Care
Lancaster University, UK

Katharina Heimerl
Associate Professor
Department of Palliative Care and Organizational Ethics
University of Klagenfurt in Vienna, Austria

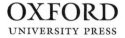
OXFORD
UNIVERSITY PRESS

OXFORD
UNIVERSITY PRESS

Great Clarendon Street, Oxford, OX2 6DP,
United Kingdom

Oxford University Press is a department of the University of Oxford.
It furthers the University's objective of excellence in research, scholarship,
and education by publishing worldwide. Oxford is a registered trade mark of
Oxford University Press in the UK and in certain other countries

First Edition published in 2013

Impression: 1

ISBN 978-0-19-964415-5

Printed and bound by
CPI Group (UK) Ltd, Croydon, CR0 4YY

Foreword

Palliative care, although still a relatively new field across medicine and other health and social care disciplines, is critical for humane end-of-life experiences, whether for a young mother dying of breast cancer, an intellectually disabled adult grappling with bereavement, an elder facing pending death, or the formal and informal care providers and organizations working with such patients and their families.

Like palliative care, action research has been something of a stepchild, not entirely accepted or prioritized by many adherents to traditional 'outside expert-driven' research traditions. An umbrella term for a spectrum of approaches that embrace participation with action and reflection as core components, action research has its deepest roots in the work of American social psychologist Kurt Lewin over 50 years ago. Yet it has only recently become more widely accepted and valued as a means of inquiry *with*, rather than *on*, communities, patients, and other groups regarding issues of deep personal relevance. With its attention to 'blurring the line' between the researchers and the researched, reducing power imbalances, building individual and community capacity, and using study findings to promote change, action research holds special relevance for fields like palliative care. Yet, to date, little work has conjoined these two areas.

In this refreshing new volume, Jo Hockley, Katherine Froggatt, and Katharina Heimerl bring together a fascinating array of chapters on action research, palliative care, and the ethical, methodological, and other issues such work entails. They and their fellow authors further present case studies that illustrate the value that is added when an action research approach is applied in work with practitioners, patients, and families to better understand and address issues and challenges related to palliative care. The case illustrations include action research in the United Kingdom, Western Europe, Australia, and North America, and span a wide range of topics. This book is not meant as an alternative to more traditional research approaches, but rather as an important supplement, and one with special relevance to the relatively uncharted territory of inquiry in palliative care. The authors' personal reflections, coupled with their accent on research that is rigorous and ethically sound, provide an excellent introduction to this important new area. Researchers, practitioners, facility administrators, and community members interested in end-of-life issues, and in studying these and other issues through a new, more participatory and action-oriented approach to inquiry, will find this book an invaluable resource.

Meredith Minkler, PhD
Professor and Director, Health and Social Behavior,
University of California, Berkeley

Preface

Jo Hockley, Katherine Froggatt,
and Katharina Heimerl

The aim of this book is to promote participatory research as an appropriate research methodology within the field of palliative care. There are many names given to the term participatory research, such as: critical action research, practitioner action research, appreciative inquiry, systemic action research, and participatory action research (PAR), to name but a few. This is best summarized by the notion of 'participatory and action-oriented approaches' (Minkler and Wallerstein, 2003). Therefore, participatory research incorporates different terms, but we hold to three core values, namely: collaboration in the research process in order to empower people, practitioners, and researchers (*participation*); to bring about change for people, organizations, and systems (*action*); and to generate knowledge through collective reflective processes (*reflection*)—all of which are incorporated in the title of this book. Throughout the book, the different terms that constitute participatory and action-oriented approaches are used interchangeably. It was not our concern to strive for one common definition or term.

Participatory research has only recently been recognized as a form of social inquiry, although its history as an approach goes back over fifty years and some would say as far back as the late nineteenth/early twentieth century to the work of Dewey (Greenwood and Levin, 1998). Whilst established within the education field, action research has more recently been used in health and social care.

This book is relevant to practitioners as well as academic researchers in palliative care. However, such a book is likely to be a challenge to health and social care professionals, and researchers, whose research has been focused within the traditional quantitative and qualitative paradigms. This is because participatory research as a methodology is unashamedly collaborative, working *with* people as co-researchers in order to change practice/organizational settings for the better. We believe that for people working within palliative care who are willing to push open a door into the world of participatory research, this book will be an important and helpful resource.

Those undertaking a participatory action research project are unlikely to be those who are faint-hearted or want a quick fix solution to problems. Instead, they are people who want to make a difference through their research to bring about change. Such change may be at the level of care for the individual/s, organization, or indeed the wider system. Within the book you will find examples of participatory research that has sought to address change at, and across, these different levels. Such research is undertaken through a more direct and collaborative way than traditional approaches allow, addressing issues of pressing concern with an emphasis on social justice.

The background of the editors reflects some of the diversity present within the action research world. We come from health backgrounds of medicine, public health, and nursing, currently working in academia and practice. Our common concern is to develop palliative care in a way that engages the people who are recipients of care as well as those providing care. In terms of research and education, palliative care is a small and relatively young discipline within healthcare (Froggatt and Hockley, 2011). Action research, similarly, is a newer research approach and therefore, like palliative care, by its presence offers a critique of the mainstream. Consequently, the field is young and many of the authors writing here are pioneers who present doctoral level research drawing upon practice backgrounds.

Overview of book

The book is divided into three sections. The chapters in Section 1 look at different theoretical frameworks or 'groundings' of participatory research. In this section, different authors make a case for the position they have adopted, with each chapter being illustrated with examples from practice. In Chapter 1, the editors give an overview of participatory research and its history, arguing its place within critical social sciences. This is taken up further in Chapter 2 where Jo Hockley places action research in the critical paradigm, giving particular attention to Habermas as cited in Kemmis (2001) as one of the critical philosophers. The use of reflexivity is highlighted as a way of bringing new knowledge to the field of end-of-life care for frail older people in nursing homes with reference to a study undertaken in the UK. In Chapter 3, Katharina Heimerl and Klaus Wegleitner describe the relevance of systems theory to participatory research. They illustrate this with their study involving organizational change in palliative care settings across the Tyrol region in Austria. They highlight the complexity of bringing about change across systems and stress the importance of valuing the individuals within such a system. Chapter 4 is a contribution from Mary Lou Kelley and Margaret McKee from Canada. They share their integrative 'community capacity development' model that is being used in participatory action research to create palliative care programmes in long-term care (LTC) homes. In Chapter 5, Geralyn Hynes expounds on first, second, and third person inquiry as a different theoretical perspective within action research. This has an important role within practice-based knowledge development. Finally in this section, Chapter 6 by Caroline Nicholson and Julie Barnes presents an account of appreciative inquiry as a participatory approach drawing upon their innovative work of people's experience of living with dementia.

Section 2 brings together exemplars of action research in palliative care across different settings, disciplines and countries. In Chapter 7, Steffen Eychmüller and Franzisca Domeisen Benedetti from Switzerland write about their experience of implementing a community-based model of palliative care provision within different regions of Switzerland and Liechtenstein. Sue Read, in Chapter 8, uses action research to promote meaningful engagement with people with intellectual disabilities within the context of loss and bereavement in the UK. Chapter 9 highlights the work by Patricia White and Marie Lynch, who used action research in a project undertaken in Ireland to develop palliative care for people with advanced respiratory disease; the study included a pathway approach across the acute general hospital, primary care, and hospice setting. Finally, in Chapter 10, Sharon Kaasalainen writes about an action-based approach to improve pain management in long-term care homes in Canada. This addresses implementation across all levels of the system.

Section 3 highlights specific issues that arise when using this uncommon but effective methodology. In Chapter 11, Sharon Andrews, Fran McInerney, and Andrew Robinson critique the issues of power that arose when undertaking a critical action research study to support change in end-of-life care within aged care facilities in Tasmania. They highlight the importance of creating understanding of power that undermine opportunities for collaboration and best practice in palliative care. Kevin Brazil writes about working together across diverse populations in Chapter 12. He draws on research with indigenous communities in Canada. He examines the ethics of participation and action research within indigenous communities coming together to undertake research to improve end-of-life care. In Chapter 13, Elisabeth Reitinger and Erich Lehner address issues of gender. They use gender analysis in action research to increase awareness of issues of power and ethics when working within Austrian organizations caring for frail older people at the end of life. Katherine Froggatt takes on the issues of rigour and quality when undertaking action research in Chapter 14. This chapter presents frameworks that can be used to evaluate the quality and rigour within projects. Sustainability of the changes in practice as a result of an action research study is highlighted in Chapter 15 by Geralyn Hynes from Ireland. Geralyn's research involved developing respiratory nursing practice to address respiratory palliative care in the acute hospital environment. She considers how cooperative inquiry, as a form of action research, offers a framework for sustaining an inquiring and problem solving approach to facilitating palliative approaches in the acute care environment. The final chapter (Chapter 16—written by the editors) draws a number of strands together by considering the challenges and opportunities in undertaking participatory research that are either set within palliative care settings or have a palliative care focus.

References

Froggatt, K. and Hockley, J. (2011) Action Research in Palliative Care: Defining an Evaluating Methodology. *Palliative Medicine*, **25**(8): 782–87.

Greenwood, D.J. and Levin, M. (1998) *Introduction to Action Research: Social Research for Social Change*. London: Sage Publications.

Kemmis, S. (2001) Exploring the Relevance of Critical Theory for Action Research: Emancipatory Action Research in the Footsteps of Jurgen Habermas. In: P. Reason and H. Bradbury (eds), *Handbook of Action Research: Participator Inquiry and Practice*, pp. 91–102. London: Sage Publications.

Minkler, M. and Wallerstein, N. (2003). Introduction to Community Based Participatory Research. In M. Minkler and N. Wallerstein (eds), *Community Based Participatory Research for Health*, pp. 3–26. San Francisco: Jossey Bass.

Acknowledgements

We would like to thank the authors who have contributed chapters to this edited book and presented insightful accounts into the complexity of action research within a palliative care context. We are conscious that these chapters represent many other people who have been willing to engage in a participatory way with important issues around palliative care. We thank them too, for, without their involvement, much change that is presented here would not have happened.

We thank the staff at Oxford University Press, including Nicola Wilson and Caroline Smith, for their support through this process.

Table of contents

List of contributors

Sharon Andrews
Wicking Dementia Research
and Education Centre,
University of Tasmania,
Tasmania, Australia

Julie Barnes
Independent Consultant/Facilitator,
UK

Kevin Brazil
School of Nursing & Midwifery,
Queen's University,
Belfast, UK

Franzisca Domeisen Benedetti
Centre for Palliative Care,
Cantonal Hospital St Gallen,
St Gallen, Switzerland

Steffen Eychmüller
Palliative Care, Inselspital Bern,
Bern, Switzerland

Katherine Froggatt
International Observatory on
End of Life Care,
Lancaster University,
Lancaster, UK

Katharina Heimerl
Department of Palliative Care
and Organizational Ethics,
University of Klagenfurt, Vienna,
Austria

Jo Hockley
St Christopher's Hospice,
London, UK

Geralyn Hynes
School of Nursing and
Midwifery, Trinity College Dublin,
Dublin, Ireland

Sharon Kaasalainen
School of Nursing,
McMaster University,
Hamilton, Canada

Mary Lou Kelley
School of Social Work,
Lakehead University,
Ontario, Canada

Erich Lehner
Department of Palliative Care
and Organizational Ethics,
University of Klagenfurt, Vienna,
Austria

Marie Lynch
Irish Hospice Foundation,
Dublin, Ireland

Fran McInerney
School of Nursing, Midwifery, and
Paramedicine, Australian Catholic
University/Mercy Health,
Melbourne, Australia

Margaret McKee
School of Social Work,
Lakehead University, Ontario, Canada

Caroline Nicholson
Florence Nightingale
School of Nursing and Midwifery,
King's College, London, UK

Sue Read
School of Nursing and Midwifery,
Keele University, Staffordshire, UK

Elisabeth Reitinger
Department of Palliative Care
and Organizational Ethics,
University of Klagenfurt, Vienna,
Austria

Andrew Robinson
School of Nursing and
Midwifery/Wicking Dementia
Research and Education Centre,
University of Tasmania,
Tasmania, Australia

Klaus Wegleitner
Department of Palliative Care
and Organizational Ethics,
University of Klagenfurt, Vienna,
Austria

Patricia White
Respiratory Assessment Unit,
St James's Hospital,
Dublin, Ireland

Anne Williams
Centre for Cancer and Palliative Care,
Perth, Australia

List of abbreviations

ACF	aged care facility		LCP	Liverpool Care Pathway
AI	appreciative inquiry		LTC	long-term care
ARG	action research group		NH	nursing home
CBPR	community based participatory research		OCAP	ownership, control, access, and possession
COPD	chronic obstructive pulmonary disease		OD	organizational development
			OPD	outpatient department
CPGs	clinical practice guidelines		PAR	participatory action research
DH	Department of Health		PCA	personal care assistant
DSU	dementia secure unit		PSW	personal support worker
EN	enrolled nurse		RACF	residential aged care facility
GSF	Gold Standard Framework		RdBGs	reflective de-briefing groups
HSE	Health Service Executive		RN	registered nurse
ID	intellectual disabilities		SCOT	strengths, challenges, opportunities, threats
IHF	Irish Hospice Foundation			
KNNPC	Kerala Neighbourhood Network in Palliative Care		UCPs	unregulated care providers
			UK	United Kingdom

Section 1

Groundings

Chapter 1

Action research: an overview

Jo Hockley, Katherine Froggatt, and
Katharina Heimerl

Introduction

Action research has only recently been recognized as a form of social inquiry. Although its history as an approach for research goes back over fifty years, and some would say as far back as the late nineteenth/early twentieth century to the work of Dewey (Greenwood and Levin, 1998), it is a more recent trend in researching practice. Prior to the mid-1980s most research in healthcare was based within the positivist or hermeneutic/interpretive paradigms. Quantitative and qualitative methodologies were often seen as 'opposed' to each other on opposite sides of the paradigm debate, but often this distinction has been overstated (Webb, 1989). With a more eclectic use of methods (Meyer, 1993) and in particular the use of 'triangulation' as a method for increasing validity in research (Webb, 1989), claims for the superiority of one paradigm over the other have decreased. Subsequently, this has increased the acceptability of practice-based research such as action research.

This chapter helps to set the scene for the following chapters in this book and outlines the history of action research as an approach to social inquiry. It defines action research and examines the philosophical perspective for those interested in using action research to research practice. Finally, this chapter challenges us within palliative care to take the necessary risks to look at our own practice and address assumptions in order that we can continue to strive for improvement in our care of people and their families facing the end of their lives.

History of action research

Action research first became popular as a research method in the USA during the 1940s/1950s. Kurt Lewin (1890–1947), a psychologist whose research was based in social and experimental psychology, is the person linked with the founding of action research. He constructed a theory concerning action research and made it a respectable research approach for social scientists (McKernan, 1991).

Lewin defined action research as a spiral of steps, each involving planning, acting, observing, and evaluating the process. These cycles involved the overlapping of action and reflection so that changes in plans were made as people learned from experience (Kemmis and McTaggart, 1988). Lewin was particularly interested that inquiry should bring about a practical improvement rather than just the writing of books: 'Research that produces nothing but books will not suffice' (Lewin, 1948: 203).

A number of other people must also take more credit for the development of action research. Jacob Moreno (1892–1974), a physician, social philosopher, and poet, who shared students with Lewin, reported the importance of integrating theory and practice by perceiving researchers as social investigators rather than just observers (Waterman *et al.*, 2001). Collier, also working in the USA, was using the terminology of action research in his work on race relations as Commissioner of Indian Affairs (1933–1945). He was convinced that: 'Since the findings of research must be carried into effect by the administrator and the layman, and must be criticized by them through their experience, the administrator and the layman must themselves participate creatively in the research impelled as it is from their own area of need' (Ebbutt, 1985: 154).

It is this emphasis on the layman's own area of need that was revolutionary as a way of research at a time when positivism was the dominant paradigm. The founding fathers of action research were interested in bringing about change in a democratic way. Some suggest that Lewin did not develop the theory of action research with respect to oppressive power bases in the context of poor manager-worker relationships (Waterman *et al.*, 2001: 1). Nonetheless, Lewin's technique of field force analysis (1952), used to identify restraining and driving forces in relation to bringing about change, highlights his awareness of the political forces within an organization. The emphasis on reducing the restraining forces is widely used in the change management of organizations, determining whether change is viable and progress can occur. Lewin died suddenly at the age of 57; for more information on the life and work of Kurt Lewin see Smith (2001).

While action research was being developed in the USA, a group of researchers in the UK were interested in using action research to underpin the work of the Tavistock Institute of Human Relations. The group was interdisciplinary, with a background in psychoanalysis and social psychology. This work has gradually evolved. It has been responsible for promoting an organizational type of action research (Burns, 2007; Coghlan and Brannick, 2001), that uses systems theory or a psycho-dynamic framework (Reason and Rowan, 1981).

From the beginnings of action research as social inquiry in education and organization development, clinical practice saw the first advocates of action research in the late 1970s (Sandow, 1979; Towell, 1979). These pioneers emphasized the importance of continually reviewing, reporting back to participants, and modification of the process in order to bring about change. The change initiatives, however, were often presented from 'top-down' management positions.

In the early to mid-1990s, there was a greater focus on understanding the theoretical position of action research in healthcare (Hart and Bond, 1996; Meyer, 1993; Titchen and Binnie, 1994). This debate continues (Reason and Bradbury, 2001), but there is greater flexibility for action researchers than in other methodologies to form research positions required to 'meet the specific conditions under which the research is to operate' (Gustavesen, 2003: 158). This will be discussed later in this chapter under philosophical perspectives of action research.

Definitions of action research

Names and definitions of action research are numerous. Most reflect the philosophical stance of those action researchers who have created them. There is a myriad of participative, experiential, and action oriented approaches to action research: appreciative inquiry; action science; participatory research; systemic action research; critical action research; cooperative inquiry; action inquiry; first person inquiry; community action research; educational action research; emancipatory research; and new paradigm research (Reason and Bradbury, 2001). Minkler and Wallerstein (2003: 5) therefore speak of 'participatory and action oriented approaches'. A comprehensive systematic review of action research by Waterman *et al.* (2001) defines action research by its inclusion of ten characteristics (see Box 1.1).

Two distinguishing features are fundamental to all approaches of action research. These are the cyclic process involving some sort of change intervention, and the partnership between researchers and practitioners. Those within practice are encouraged to identify the difficulties that they want to research, and, together with the researcher, come up with ideas to help overcome the problems.

Greenwood (1994) has argued that the two main purposes of action research are to implement change and to generate theory. One could also argue that what needs to be made explicit about action research is the importance of critical self-reflection. Unless practitioners are encouraged to critically reflect on practice, it is unlikely that practice will change.

Box 1.1 Ten characteristics of action research (Waterman *et al.*, 2001).

- ◆ AR describes, interprets, and explains social situations.
- ◆ AR incorporates a change intervention aimed at improvement.
- ◆ AR is problem-focused, context-specific, and future-orientated.
- ◆ AR is a group activity—partnership between action researcher/s and participants.
- ◆ AR is educative and empowering.
- ◆ AR is dynamic, involving cycles of: problem identification, planning, action, and evaluation.
- ◆ AR uses reflection as a way of learning about situations and issues.
- ◆ AR uses both qualitative and quantitative research methods to collect data.
- ◆ AR acquires both practical and prepositional knowledge.
- ◆ AR is able to validate old theories and/or generate new theories from practice.

Data from McNiff and Whitehead, *All You Need to Know About Action Research*, SAGE Publications Ltd, London, UK, copyright © 2006.

The following definition of action research is much used:

> Action research is a participatory, democratic process concerned with developing practical knowing in the pursuit of worthwhile human purposes, grounded in a participatory worldview which we believe is emerging at this historical moment. It seeks to bring together action and reflection, theory and practice, in participation with others, in the pursuit of practical solutions to issues of pressing concern to people, and more generally the flourishing of individual persons their communities.
>
> (Reason and Bradbury, 2001: 1)

The collaborative nature of action research is evident from the fact that it is not research 'on' people, nor is it research 'for' people, but research 'with' people (Reason and Bradbury, 2001). Meyer (2000), in quoting from the seminal work by Carr and Kemmis (1986), simply suggests that action research incorporates three important characteristics: it is participatory, it is democratic, and it contributes to social change and social theory.

Philosophical perspectives and action research

There has been considerable debate in the literature as to where action research is positioned within the three classical paradigms of research (quantitative/positivist, qualitative/interpretive, and critical theory) (see Figure 1.1). McKernan (1991), an educationalist, aligned models of action research across the three classical research paradigms, namely: the scientific-technical view of problem-solving used by Lewin within his experimental group work of the early twentieth century; the

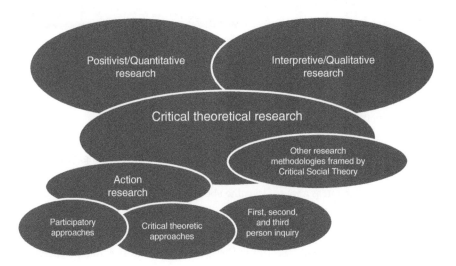

Fig. 1.1 Action research and its position within the research paradigms.
Adapted with permission from McNiff and Whitehead, *Action Research: Principles and Practice*, Second Edition, Routledge Farmer, London, copyright © 2006.

practical-deliberative approach, where 'the action research develops a personal inter-pretive understanding from working on practical problems' (Elliott, 1987: 157); and finally, the critical-emancipatory paradigm for educational action research. It is this latter stance that is argued by educationalists Carr and Kemmis (1986), as well as McNiff and Whitehead (2002), as being the only possible approach if those within practice are to be empowered to change.

Holter and Schwartz-Barcott (1993) also name three action research approaches: the 'technical collaborative' approach; the 'mutual collaborative' approach; and the 'enhancement' approach. However, unlike McKernan, the different approaches are firmly based within critical theory because of their participatory/collaborative nature. They align the approaches with critical theorist Habermas (1972) and his the-ory of knowledge-constitutive interests. Meyer and Batehup (1997) agree with many in the paradigm debate of action research that the positivist and interpretive paradigms are inappropriate, as Carr and Kemmis (1986) highlight: 'Both the interpretive approach and positivist approach convey a similar understanding of educational researchers and of the relationship to the research act. In both approaches, the researcher stands outside the researched situation adopting a disinterested stance in which any explicit concern with critically evaluating and changing the educational realities being analysed is rejected' (Carr and Kemmis, 1986: 99).

Greenwood (1994), from within nursing, cautions using a critical approach to action research suggesting that although there might be similarities between the professions of teaching and nursing, nursing does not boast such an autonomous position in practice as does classroom teaching. Nursing is bound up with colleagues from different disci-plines and may therefore be exposed to more powerful healthcare professionals/managers when it comes to bringing about change. Even so, the emphasis on under-standing power issues is a vital aspect of critical social science (see Chapters 2 and 11).

Amidst all the debate about which philosophical paradigm is most suitable for action research, Hart and Bond (1995; 1996) devised a typology specifically for health and social care, categorizing different types of action research in order to clarify the complexity of different approaches. The four types track the historical progression of action research as a strategy, from the experimental work of Lewin through to feminist approaches within social communities:

- The *experimental type* that arose out of Lewin's original scientific work in group dynamics.
- The *organizational type* developed by Emery and Trist (1965), colleagues at the Tavistock Institute during the 1960s and 1970s, who recognized that the traditional way of organizing work from the top down was hierarchical and not open to debate—a closed system—which participation in action research challenged.
- The *professionalizing type* that has been associated with education and healthcare.
- The *empowering type* that has developed through social communities.

Hart and Bond (1995) state that the different types of action research as detailed above may be highlighted at differing stages in any one action research project. They argue that a study is thus capable of moving along the continuum from a consensus to a conflict model of society. The *experimental approach* would be positioned at the consensus end, with the *empowering* approach at the conflict end. However, being eclectic and drawing on the different approaches of action research as suggested by Hart and Bond (1995) requires considerable knowledge and experience of action research. Waterman *et al.* (2001) attempted to use Hart and Bond's typology to categorize studies in a systematic review of action research but found it 'did not accurately reflect the findings in the included studies' (Waterman *et al.*, 2001: 11).

We would like to support ideas from the work of McNiff and Whitehead (2002), who suggest that different approaches to action research can be accommodated within the critical social paradigm (see again Figure 1.1). They highlight that action research is about the involvement of others in the field, and researching practice together in order to bring about change. Such a stance within research does not fit the philosophical slant of the positivist and interpretive research. Action research is about empowerment and working with those within the field to bring about change. It is therefore appropriate that whatever action research approach is used it is important to see its emergence through the critical theoretical paradigm. It may be that we are at quite a 'historical moment' in the whole paradigm debate, as insightfully suggested by Reason and Bradbury (2001: 1) in their definition of action research cited earlier in this chapter. Certainly McNiff and Whitehead (2006: 41) point out that critical theory asks: 'How can this situation be understood in order to change it?' whereas action research goes further and asks: 'How can it be changed?'.

Whatever the debate, action research is not for the faint-hearted! Gummesson (2000: 116) has called it 'the most demanding and far-reaching method of doing case study research'. The involvement with others in the field, and the emphasis on researching practice in order to bring about change makes action research more complex than its name might imply (Waterman *et al.*, 2001). Meyer (2000) stresses that the success of any action research should not necessarily be judged by the size of change resulting from it, but rather 'in relation to what has been learnt from the experience of undertaking the work' (Meyer, 2000: 180).

Ways of knowing and the adopted worldview when undertaking action research: the epistemology and ontology of action research

A fundamental aspect of action research is the importance of gaining knowledge from practice (Holter and Schwartz-Barcott, 1993; Meyer, 2000; Williamson *et al.*, 2012). How we come to judge what credible knowledge is, involves understanding what we mean by knowledge and whether practical knowledge is in fact 'scientific'. Those from a positivist paradigm would see knowledge (epistemology): 'as a free-standing unit, with an existence of its own, residing "out there" in books and databases. In this view, knowledge is divorced from the people who create it' (McNiff and Whitehead, 2002: 18).

Action researchers do not believe in there being only one way of knowing things. Instead they understand the generation of knowledge to occur as a result of many ways of being in the world (McNiff and Whitehead, 2002). Knowledge is rooted in the experience of 'doing' (Ladkin, 2004). Action researchers in particular derive knowledge collaboratively with those involved in practice.

Theoretical knowledge traditionally has held a more superior position than practice knowledge. However, Benner (1984) stresses the importance of tacit or commonsense knowledge that comes from experience as a way of learning. It was John Dewey, the philosopher/teacher who first drew attention to the importance of experiential knowledge: 'We learn by doing and realizing what came of what we did' (Dewey, 1938—cited in Rolf *et al.*, 2001: 2). One of the ways to get at knowledge about what one is doing (experiential or tacit knowledge) is through actively reflecting on specific situations in order to understand and critically analyse them.

Those undertaking action research adopt a way of being (ontological perspective) that is very different from those using the positivist/interpretive paradigm. In order to get at the tacit knowledge that underpins practice, action researchers build relationships with practitioners and adopt them as co-researchers. Action researchers help collaborators from within practice to question and critically reflect on the values that underpin their practice (Nolan and Grant, 1993). Action researchers themselves are used as part of the change mechanism; their research therefore is not value-free but will inevitably be tied up with their own previous experience alongside that of co-researchers in the project from within the clinical setting. They see themselves working in partnership with people within practice in order to bring about change. See Table 1.1 for a collation of the epistemology, ontology, and methodology of action research collated from McNiff and Whitehead (2006).

Table 1.1 The stance from which researchers view knowledge and the adopted worldview when undertaking action research

	The perspective when undertaking action research
Epistemology (how we understand knowledge)	◆ Knowledge is not out there with an independent existence. ◆ Knowledge is generated from experience of living and learning. ◆ Knowledge is a living process and therefore will always need adding to. ◆ Knowledge creation involves social processes and can only be provisional as subject to others interpretation and critique.
Ontology (how we view the world)	◆ Accommodates multiple perspectives. ◆ Values based on inclusiveness and building of relationships. ◆ Recognition of place of 'I' in research. ◆ Underpinned by social justice with respect for pluralistic forms. ◆ Commitment to action within the research process.
Methodology (how we do research)	◆ Participatory and collaborative. ◆ Shows cycles of action and reflection. ◆ Demonstrates relationships of influence. ◆ Focus is 'open-ended' and developmental. ◆ The aim is to improve learning in order to improve social practices.

Data from McNiff and Whitehead, *Action Research: Principles and Practice*, Second Edition, Routledge Farmer, London, copyright © 2006.

Action research revolves around the cycle of observing/diagnosing, reflecting/ planning, taking action, evaluating that action, and then modifying prior to a further cycle. It is known as the action-reflection cycle (Coghlan and Brannick, 2001; McNiff and Whitehead, 2006: 9). Criticism regarding rigour and action research can be levied at action researchers from those whose research is based in the positivist and interpretive paradigms. It is important therefore to report the different cycles of action and how one's own assumptions were challenged while undertaking the study. Coghlan and Brannick (2001: 24) maintain that a good action research project contains three main aims, namely: a good story of what happened; a rigorous reflection on that story in order to make sense of it; an extrapolation of usable knowledge or theory from reflection on the story.

Action research is conducted by practitioners alongside co-researchers who are prepared to challenge the status quo. Practitioners are helped to ask why things are as they are and what they feel needs changing for the better. In many ways it requires action researchers to be quite entrepreneurial in their readiness to think creatively. There are three attributes to action research that run across the many different approaches that we will see reported in this book. First, approaches of action research are always participatory although the level of participation in any one study can vary. The more confident the action researcher or the better they are supported by experienced action researchers, the greater the level of participation in the research. Second, action research is a practice-based approach to research that is fundamentally an agent of change. And finally, evidence collected within an action research study challenges 'taken for granted' assumptions from within everyday practice (see Chapter 5).

The underlying ethos of action research is summarized by Burns (2007: 13) in the following:

- It combines a systematic study, sometimes experimental, of a social problem as well as endeavouring to solve it.

- It includes a spiral process of data collation to determine goals and assessment of the results of intervention.

- It demands feedback of the results of intervention to all parties involved in the research.

- It implies continuous cooperation between researchers and practitioners.

- It relies on the principles of group dynamics and is anchored in its change phases. The phases are unfreezing, moving, and refreezing. Decision making is mutual and is carried out in a public way.

- It takes into account issues of values, objectives, and the power needs of the parties involved.

- It serves to create knowledge, to formulate principles of intervention and also to develop instruments for selection, intervention, and training.

- Within the framework of action research there is much emphasis on recruitment, training, and support of the change agents.

When these positions are properly adopted within projects there is an exciting simultaneous contribution to change in practice as well as an addition to social science knowledge. In our increasingly postmodern culture, we believe that tacit knowledge is central to understanding within any one culture.

Palliative care and action research

The UK Hospice Movement emerged in the mid-1960s as a result of Dame Cicely Saunders' work at St Christopher's Hospice, London. There was, however, interest already growing outside the UK, and soon a worldwide network was set up with particular collaboration in the late 1970s between the USA, Canada, India, and Australia. The term 'palliative care' was adopted shortly after and was derived from the Latin word *palliare*, meaning 'to cloak'; the fact that the cancer could no longer be cured meant this was put to one side in favour of the holistic care needs of the patient and family (Davies and Seymour, 2002).

Palliative care has developed differently in many countries across the world and has often depended on a country's specific culture/context in how the concept has been introduced. In the UK, palliative medicine became a specialty in 1986, encouraging the teaching of palliative care within the medical curriculum and the formation of training posts within specialist palliative care units (Davies and Seymour, 2002). This encouraged the generation of hospital-based palliative care teams with the dissemination of knowledge about palliative care being accepted and advocated in the settings where the majority of people were dying (Hockley and Dunlop, 1998).

It has only been since the late 1990s that there has been a greater emphasis on applying knowledge developed within specialist palliative care to other diseases and in other settings. As a result of this, the definition of palliative care has become more inclusive of diseases other than cancer: 'An approach that improves the quality of life of patients and their families facing the problems associated with life-threatening illness, through the prevention and relief of suffering by means of early identification and impeccable assessment and treatment of pain and other problems, physical, psychosocial and spiritual' (Sepulveda *et al.*, 2002: 94).

It is exciting that a majority of the chapters in this book represent this dissemination of specialist palliative care to the generalist setting. Many of the projects cited are about the development of palliative care services for patients with chronic diseases, persons with disabilities, as well as older persons and persons with dementia, rather than cancer. Interestingly, however, we have found it difficult to locate many specialist palliative care centres undertaking action research projects. We asked ourselves 'why this might be?' It is certainly not the case that the specialty of palliative care is not undertaking research—there is plenty of research into symptom control and the experience of different aspects of end-of-life care from both patients and their families. However, actually researching day-to-day practice within specialist palliative care using an action research approach is much less common. We do hope that there is not a sense of disappointment by the lack of examples of action research from within specialist palliative care; instead we hope that any disappointment might become the fuel for ideas for such a project. Perhaps the creative interest that led to the emergence of the hospice movement some fifty years ago now needs to be risked.

Conclusion

This chapter has provided an overview of action research: its historical roots within organizational action research, through education, and now into healthcare research. It has described the many approaches to action research and provided an argument for action research developing out of critical theory.

In this book there are not examples from each approach, but we hope there is a good enough selection to open the door to action research and its possibilities within practice-based palliative care research and even specialist palliative care. In order to stay ahead of the changing world that any one organization faces, it is important to adopt a flexible enough approach to consider different research methodologies for different research projects. As editors we would like, with this book, to pose action research as a very important research approach for palliative care in order to confront our assumptions about our care of patients and their families and to continue to advance end-of-life care practice for the better.

References

Benner, P. (1984) *From Novice to Expert: Excellence and Power in Clinical Nursing Practice.* Menlo Park, CA: Addison-Wesley.

Burns, D. (2007) *Systemic Action Research: A Strategy for Whole System Change.* Bristol: The Policy Press.

Carr, W. and Kemmis, S. (1986) *Becoming Critical: Education, Knowledge and Action Research.* London: The Falmer Press.

Coghlan, D. and Brannick, T. (2001) *Doing Action Research in Your Own Organization.* London: Sage Publications Ltd.

Davies, S. and Seymour, J. (2002) Historical and Policy Contexts. In: J. Hockley and D. Clark (eds), *Palliative Care for Older People in Care Homes*, pp. 4–33. Oxford: Oxford University Press.

Ebbutt, D. (1985) Educational Action Research: Some General Concerns and Specific Quibbles. In: R. Burgess (ed.), *Issues in Educational Research*, pp. 152–74. Lewes: Falmer.

Elliott, J. (1987) Educational Theory, Practical Philosophy and Action Research. *British Journal of Educational Studies*, **25**: 149–69.

Emery, F.E. and Trist, E.L. (1965) The Causal Texture of Organizational Environments. *Human Relations*, **18**: 21–32.

Greenwood, J. (1994) Action Research: A Few Details, A Caution and Something New. *Journal of Advanced Nursing*, **20**: 13–18.

Greenwood, D.J. and Levin, M. (1998) *Introduction to Action Research.* London: Sage Publications.

Gummesson, E. (2000) *Qualitative Methods in Management Research*, 2nd edn. California: Thousand Oaks.

Gustavsen, B. (2003) New Forms of Knowledge Production and The Role of Action Research. *Action Research*, **1**(2): 153–64.

Habermas, J. (1972) *Knowledge and Human Interest* (translated by Jeremy J. Shapiro). London: Heinemann Educational.

Hart, E. and Bond, M. (1995) *Action Research for Health and Social Care: a Guide to Practice.* Buckingham: Open University Press.

Hart, E. and Bond, M. (1996) Making Sense of Action Research Through the Use of a Typology. *Journal of Advanced Nursing*, **23**: 152–9.

Hockley, J. and Dunlop, R. (1998) *Hospital-based Palliative Care Teams: the Hospital/Hospice Interface*. Oxford: Oxford University Press.

Holter, I. and Schwartz-Barcott, D. (1993) Action Research: What is it? How Has it Been Used and How Can it Be Used in Nursing? *Journal of Advanced Nursing*, **18**: 298–304.

Kemmis, S. and McTaggart, R. (1988) *The Action Research Planner*. Deakin: Deakin University Press.

Ladkin, D. (2004) Action Research in Practice: What the Books Don't Tell You. In: C. Seale, G. Gobo, J.F. Gubrium, and D. Silverman (eds), *Qualitative Research Practice*, pp. 536–48. London: Sage Publications.

Lewin, K. (1948) *Resolving Social Conflicts*. New York: Harper.

Lewin, K. (1952) *Field Theory in Social Science*. London: Tavistock.

McKernan. J. (1991) *Curriculum Action Research: a Handbook of Methods and Resources for the Reflective Practitioner*. London: Kogan Page Ltd.

McNiff, J. and Whitehead, J. (2002) *Action Research: Principles and Practice*, 2nd edn. London: RoutledgeFalmer.

McNiff, J. and Whitehead, J. (2006) *All You Need to Know About Action Research*. London: Sage.

Meyer, J. (1993) New Paradigm Research in Practice: The Trials and Tribulations of Action Research. *Journal of Advanced Nursing*, **18**: 1066–72.

Meyer, J. (2000) Using Qualitative Methods in Health Related Action Research. *British Medical Journal*, **320**: 178–81.

Meyer, J. and Batehup, L. (1997) Action Research in Health-Care Practice: Nature, Present Concerns and Future Possibilities. *NTresearch*, **2**(3): 175–84.

Minkler, M. and Wallerstein, N. (2003) Introduction to Community Based Participatory Research. In: M. Minkler and N. Wallerstein (eds), *Community Based Participatory Research for Health*, pp. 3–26. San Francisco: Jossey Bass.

Nolan, M. and Grant, G. (1993) Action Research and Quality of Care: A Mechanism for Agreeing Basic Values as a Precursor to Change. *Journal of Advanced Nursing*, **18**: 305–311.

Reason, P. and Bradbury, H. (2001) Introduction: Inquiry and Participation in Search of a World Worthy of Human Aspiration. In: P. Reason and H. Bradbury (eds), *Handbook of Action Research: Participative Inquiry and Practice*, pp. 1–14. London: Sage Publications.

Reason, P. and Rowan, J. (eds) (1981) *Human Inquiry: A Sourcebook of New Paradigm Research*. Chichester: John Wiley.

Rolfe, G., Freshwate, D., and Jasper, M. (2001) *Critical Reflection for Nursing and the Helping Professions: A User's Guide*. London: Palgrave Macmillan.

Sandow, S. (1979) Action Research and Evaluation: Can Research and Practice be Successfully Combined? *Child: Health, Care and Development*, **5**(3): 211–23.

Sepulveda, C., Marlin, A., Yoshida, T., and Ullrich, A. (2002) Palliative Care: The World Health Organization's Global Perspective. *Journal of Pain and Symptom Control*, **24**(2): 91–6.

Smith, M.K. (2001) Kurt Lewin, Groups, Experiential Learning and Action Research. *The Encyclopedia of Informal Education*: http://www.infed.org/thinkers/et-lewin.htm (accessed 3 November 2011).

Titchen, A. and Binnie, A. (1994) Action research: a Strategy for Theory Generation and Testing. *International Journal of Nursing Studies*, **31**(1): 1–12.

Towell, D. (1979) A 'Social Systems' Approach to Research and Change in Nursing Care. *Journal of Nursing Studies*, **16**(1): 111–21.

Waterman, H., Tillen, D., Dickson, R., and de Koning, R. (2001) *Action Research: A Systematic Review and Guidance for Assessment*. Copies available from: The National Coordinating Centre for Health Technology Assessment, Southampton SO16 7PX. http://nww.hta. hnsweb.nhs.uk.

Webb, C. (1989) Action Research: Philosophy, Methods and Personal Experiences. *Journal of Advanced Nursing*, **14**: 403–10.

Williamson, G., Bellman, L., and Webster, J. (2012) *Action Research in Nursing and Healthcare*. London: Sage.

Chapter 2

Critical theory and action research

Jo Hockley

There has been considerable debate in the literature as to where action research is positioned within the classical research paradigms of the social sciences. This chapter furthers the discussion commenced in Chapter 1, where we placed action research within the critical social theory paradigm.

In this chapter I will first outline critical social theory in relation to action research, and then link reflection and action, and theory and practice as important elements of a critical approach. Finally, the chapter illustrates a critical action research study (Hockley, 2006; Hockley and Froggatt, 2006) undertaken in two UK nursing care homes. Space is made to reflect on specific aspects of action research that became apparent while undertaking the study, namely: co-researchers in action research; issues of power and authority; and critically linking theory to practice when bringing about change.

An outline of critical social theory in relation to action research

Critical social theory can best be understood from the perspective of 'the empowerment of individuals in an attempt to confront the injustice of a particular society or sphere within the society' (Kincheloe and McLaren, 1994: 140). It is concerned with bringing about improvement in the human condition. Kincheloe and McLaren define critical theory in broad terms where:

> All thought is fundamentally mediated by power relations that are socially and historically constituted; … facts can never be isolated from the domain of values; … relationships between concept and object are never stable or fixed and often mediated by the social relations of capitalist production and consumption; … certain groups in any society are privileged over others; … oppression is most forcefully reproduced when subordinates accept their social status; … language is central to the formation of subjectivity; … mainstream research practices are generally, although most unwittingly, implicated in the reproduction of systems of class, race, and gender oppression.
>
> (Kincheloe and McLaren, 1994: 139)

Critical social theory and its development within the Frankfurt School of social scientists is complex but well expounded by Held (1980). There were two distinct generations of critical social theorists, but all were concerned about the dominance of positivist science: 'Philosophers have only interpreted the world, in various ways; the point is to change it' (Marx, 1845: XI). Although Marxist thought is often viewed as 'revolutionary', one main principle which underpinned his thought, and remains a core theme for critical social theory, is the encouragement of individuals, whatever their job within an organization/society, to have a voice to shape that society. We need to remind ourselves that this is a principle that underpins democracy.

As one of the second generation critical theorists, Habermas (1972) in his thesis on *Knowledge and Human Interest*, believed that there were three levels of thinking in which knowledge became important to human beings for situations to be changed. These were: 'Information that expands our power of technical control; interpretations that make possible the orientation of action within common traditions; and analyses that free consciousness from its dependence on hypostatized powers' (Habermas, 1972: 313).

Habermas believes that change in society occurs by stressing the importance of critical self-reflection and acting responsibly on that reflection, in the interest of others. It is this use of self-reflection that emphasizes the ability of a human being to adapt to situations, balancing the intuitive nature concerning action along with what is considered to be for the good of a democratic society. For Habermas, the composition of knowledge about something, and the human interest in it, are categorized through the intermediary of work, language, and power. It is the ability of human beings to critique what is going on around them (e.g. through self-reflection and dialogue) that overcomes the egoistic self-centredness of human beings. For Habermas, true self-reflection on the object and subject of knowledge in light of human interest meant that there was potential for the greater good within a society. Of course, this can sound utopian; there are people who not only feel but also are disempowered.

Carr and Kemmis (1986) have more recently taken up the mantle of critical theory to provide an overarching philosophical framework for action research. They emphasize the importance of critical questioning within postmodern society and research which traditionally has not been possible within the positivist and interpretive paradigms.

> For any reduction of the social sciences to the explication of subjective meanings fails to recognize that the subjective meanings that characterize social life are themselves conditioned by an objective context that limits both the scope of individuals' intentions and the possibility of their realization. By adopting an epistemology for the process of self-understanding that excludes critically questioning the content of such understanding, the interpretive approach cannot assess the extent to which any existing forms of communication may be systematically distorted by prevailing social, cultural or political conditions.
>
> (Carr and Kemmis, 1986: 135)

To this end, Kemmis (2001) highlights the importance of considering action research within a critical social science paradigm and within a Habermasian critique in particular, using as his main argument Habermas's theses on *Theory of Communicative Action* (Habermas, 1984; 1987). Habermas's interest in democracy, and the importance of dialogue and action in order to overcome difficulties within society, is the basis of these theses. Habermas conceptualizes modern society as having two equal perspectives: the 'system' in which we live and, the 'lifeworld' of the people as an integral part of that system. For Habermas the 'system' is portrayed as the economic system of capitalism. In his theory, the increasingly complex manner in which the capitalist state operates means that the 'system' becomes increasingly autonomous, with potentially less and less of a human element within that system. Habermas criticises Parsons' thesis on social systems where the 'lifeworld' of people within the system is marginalized as part of a sub-system. Habermas (1987a) believes that the 'lifeworld' is much more vital and argues for the importance of the 'lifeworld' as having a value on a par with the 'system'. 'The overall task of a critical social science, including critical action research is to explore and address the interconnections and tensions between system and lifeworld aspects of a setting as they are lived out in practice' (Kemmis, 2001: 98).

An important part of action research therefore is the emphasis on creating a space/dialogue that involves representatives from across an organization. Inevitably, there are tensions within any organization; however, a key lever to bringing about successful change is enabling people within the organization to feel valued enough so that their voice is heard and debated. Bringing about this 'communicative space' (Kemmis, 2001) across an organization in order for individual voices to be heard is an important starting point for dialogue. It helps to defuse the often powerful voice of management in order to achieve mutual understanding and coming to a consensus about how things should be taken forward.

People have the ability to understand complex situations, and because of this are able to discuss and reconcile difficult situations in order to bring about change. Change does not just happen; it requires negotiation between the differing parties involved.

Despite some critics (Webb, 1996), there is an increasing interest in a critical theoretic approach to action research from those within healthcare management, nurse education, and practice (Holter and Schwartz-Barcott, 1993; Manley, 2000; 2001; Titchen, 2000; Williamson *et al.*, 2012). Bellman (1999) successfully developed patient self-medication, patient information leaflets, and patient-controlled analgesia in a surgical ward. In her thesis, she explores and exposes political dimensions of organizational culture, power, and control. Manley (2001) used critical action research to highlight the importance of the nurse consultant role in the transforming of nursing practice.

Linking reflection and action within critical action research

Critical theory can be seen as a reflexive methodology (Alvesson and Skoldberg, 2000) within which critical reflection plays a key part in the interpretation of social situations. Critical reflection and its interpretation are about uncovering the 'unconscious processes, ideologies, power relations, and other expressions of dominance that entail the privileging of certain interests over others' (Alvesson and Skoldberg, 2000: 144).

Reflection as part of action research is therefore an intensely political endeavour (Kemmis, 1985) and not just a personal encounter. If as a result of reflecting together something needs changing, then such a change must be communicated to the rest of the organization. How that communication occurs, and the willingness with which it is listened to, can make or break an action research study. Reflection therefore is not just the prerogative of the action researcher and a few interested people. Reflection is for all of those collaborating to bring about change. Because of this, the importance of management and not just practitioners being part of a reflective space is fundamental to the process of change.

Rolfe *et al.* (2001) argue for the importance of such reflection, not only to bring about critical understanding of a situation (see also Chapter 11) but also to bring about appropriate learning in order to change individual practice with the aim of influencing the culture of the practice setting. Critical reflection therefore is 'meta-thinking' (Kemmis, 1985), where thinking about thinking takes place, and the relationship between thoughts and actions is worked out. This is expanded further in Chapter 5 where first, second, and third person inquiry is discussed.

In a study that I will outline later in this chapter, enabling staff in two nursing homes to reflect not only on their practice but also on the context (i.e. the nursing home organization and its culture) was an important part of the study. Staff were encouraged to clarify difficulties in end-of-life care through reflection, and to think through solutions. This not only brought about change in the immediate situation but also added to my understanding and the body of theoretical knowledge involved in caring for older people dying in nursing homes (Hockley, 2002). This new knowledge helped to bridge the gap between theory and practice.

Linking theory and practice in critical action research

Bridging what is seen as the theory/practice gap is increasingly debated in academic literature. Some believe that this theory/practice gap needs closing (Rolfe, 1993; 1997), while others strongly believe that this perceived gap adds a creative tension which enables clinical practice to be focused and up to date (Rafferty *et al.*, 1996). Whether it needs closing or not, it is only by being involved as researchers with practitioners that knowledge about practice can be theorized and developed dialectically alongside practitioners. Bringing together theory and practice through reflection is a main feature of 'praxis' in action research (Williamson *et al.*, 2012).

Praxis is not a new concept. Its roots are found as far back as the writings of Aristotle in the third century BC. More recently, 'praxis' has been associated with critical theorists such as Habermas (1974) and Freire (1970) (see Chapter 12 for more about Freire's philosophical approach).

Rolfe (1993: 176) defines praxis as the 'bringing together of theory and practice involving a continual process of hypothesizing and testing out of new ideas, and [then] modifying practice according to the results'. Praxis is knowing 'why' we do something. It is reflecting on why something happened, in order to bring to the surface an explanation of what occurred and what could have been done to bring about a better outcome or what was done that created such a good outcome. It is not static like technical knowledge. Bringing together practice and theory through reflection helps to advance learning.

Rolfe *et al.* (2001) believe that acquiring experiential theoretical knowledge through critical reflection can create informal theory—theory that is acquired from practice.

Whereas traditional theory is applied to practice, 'informal theory' is constructed from practice (Rolfe, 1997). Holter and Schwartz-Barcott (1993) highlight that action research helps not only to bridge the gap between theory and practice but between theory, practice, and research.

There is a danger that the focus of action research can concentrate too much on action and not enough on the research aspects of the study (Meyer and Batehup, 1997). A greater critical approach to the process of change, not only from the researcher/s but also from the practitioners, is an important way of theorizing about action research within any project and the change that the context and people are undergoing.

I will now illustrate by way of reflecting critically on a piece of critical action research that was undertaken between 2000 and 2003. I will draw on some of the points discussed in the previous sections as part of my reflection.

The application of critical action research in developing end-of-life care with staff in two nursing homes

Up until the turn of the 21st century, very little palliative care research in the care of frail older people living in nursing homes in the United Kingdom had been undertaken. However, Froggatt (2000) had carried out an evaluation of a palliative care educational programme for 57 nursing homes in the north-west of England. In her research she identified that after six months of following the educational programme there was little change in practice back in the nursing homes. Staff had been enthusiastic about the course but did not have the power to bring about the changes they would have liked. For me, this study became a platform for choosing a critical action research methodology to help me understand the difficulties of bringing about that change, and to help staff think through solutions in order to develop a structure for high quality end-of-life care in two volunteering nursing homes (Hockley, 2006). Not only would there be an opportunity to work with staff to help them think about their practice caring for frail older people at the end of life, but it would also give me greater understanding of some of the issues which could be used to add to the knowledge concerning frail older people requiring generalist palliative care.

The study (Hockley, 2006; Hockley and Froggatt, 2006) is briefly described in Box 2.1. In the style of critical action research, I have reflected on the process of using such a methodology highlighting three specific components of critical action research, namely: participation; power and authority; and, adding to theory while bringing about change.

Issues of participation

One could argue that staff participation in the exploratory phase, especially in NH1, had been passive. Staff had been involved in focus groups and interviews but none had taken the role as co-researchers with me. I realized that there were probably a couple of reasons why this was the case. In reading much of the literature, I had oversimplified the 'observe, plan, act, and reflect' cycle (Kemmis and McTaggart, 1988; Stringer, 1996). I had not realized the importance of participation alongside all aspects of this cycle. Second, I felt the need to perform as a researcher in front of the owners and

Box 2.1 Outline of the critical action project (Hockley, 2006).

Phase 1 (exploratory phase): This phase ran for four months in the first nursing home (NH1) and three months in the second nursing home (NH2). It explored the NH contexts as a place where frail, older people died. I worked alongside staff caring for the frailest residents in the NHs two days/week in a research position as an outsider/insider. This gave me an opportunity to get to know the staff, who in turn supported the research. Collection of data included using: focus groups with staff; interviews with nurse managers and general practitioners; observational data recorded in a reflective diary; and documentary evidence recorded in relation to end-of-life care. Analyses of data were fed back formally and informally. While data revealed good aspects concerning physical care, it highlighted 'context' and 'clinical' issues in relation to end-of-life care, namely: time constraints and low morale amongst staff; a task orientated culture that lacked a culture of learning; closed communication culture around death and dying; a lack of psycho-social care and lack of knowledge about symptom control; and, imminent dying was not recognized. The overriding theme emphasized that the functional rehabilitative care focus of the nursing homes, with an emphasis on striving to keep alive, made dying peripheral to the care home culture.

Phase 2 (facilitative phase): Data was fed back at an open meeting with staff, management, and owners in both NHs. In NH1, staff and management requested end-of-life education and a decision made to reflect together following a death. Action 1 was the implementation of reflective de-briefing groups (RdBGs)—following a request from night staff these were then recorded. The RdBGs became an important time of communication, support and dialogue as well as a time for opportunistic learning. In NH2, as well as the RdBGs care staff also requested formulating a tool to guide care before a resident died. Staff felt there were so many things to think about, such as symptom control, psycho-social care, and care of the family. With permission, the Liverpool Care Pathway for the Dying (Ellershaw and Wilkinson, 2003) was adapted to the NH context by a small group including: the local general practitioner; care staff and nurses; NH managers; and a representative from the local regulatory body. This process and its implementation became Action 2.

Phase 3 (evaluation phase): The summative evaluation included formative evaluations as a result of changes within the NHs alongside the evaluation of the two main actions through a questionnaire to staff, and interviews with relatives and nurse managers. The RdBGs highlighted three core functions: an educative function; a supportive function; and a communicative function. The educative function was seen to have three different levels (being taught; developing understanding; critically thinking when staff challenged peers). The communicative function enabled staff within the NHs to come together to discuss how each felt about the death, what went well, and what care needed changing. The supportive function highlighted the opportunity for staff to share thoughts concerning a resident's death and its impact on them.

Staff found that the adapted Liverpool Care Pathway (LCP) documentation helped clarify complex situations and acted as a reminder. They also found it very inclusive helping team relationships and communication with the family. Families reported their satisfaction, saying 'that so much was being done in the last days of life'. Difficulties included: the need for training; time required to commence the LCP; and the wording required further simplification to enable full understanding for both care assistants and nurses using the documentation.

Reproduced from Hockley, J. (2006) *Developing High Quality End-of-life Care in Nursing Care Homes: An Action Research Study*, with permission of the author.

APPLICATION OF CRITICAL ACTION RESEARCH

nurse manager of NH1. Much of this could have been self-generated because of a degree of insecurity in what was an unpredictable methodology. But there was an obvious scrutiny of 'what I was up to'. I could have been more participative with the nurse manager in NH1 rather than just with staff. However, the pressure on her time, much of which was taken up with her commitment to excellent physical care and reporting on a daily basis to the owners, meant time for the action research study became eroded. There was an expectation that the research was my business and at the early stages of the inquiry I was content with this. I had missed the opportunity for opening up a 'communicative space' at the beginning of the study.

When it came to feeding back data from the exploratory phase, my outsider/insider position as an action researcher (see Chapters 12 and 15) was highlighted. Titchen and Binnie (1993: 859) report 'tension between the researcher and the actors in the outsider model of action research'. However, there had been advantages of being an outsider as I was able to be naive about the culture which had helped me understand important differences between the nursing home context and that of the hospice (see Hockley, 2002). But I was not prepared for the reaction to feeding back data from the exploratory phase with a formal report to management prior to feeding back informally to all staff. The written feedback provoked a strong reaction from the owners of NH1 and the nurse manager, despite previously good meetings. The feedback highlighted the excellent physical care of residents and the keenness of many staff for quality end-of-life care. It was the aligning some of the end-of-life clinical issues with the context of the NH that was not welcomed. Interestingly, there was no criticism regarding the end-of-life care issues raised. My outsider position in the action research process was highlighted and I was told it was not for me to comment on how care was managed in the home even though it influenced end-of-life care.

Meyer (2000) highlights the importance of trust when outsiders work with practitioners within an organization. From the beginning it appeared that trust had developed very easily with the care staff. Even with the owners of NH1 and the nurse manager, there did not appear to be a lack of trust prior to presenting the formal feedback. Feeding back the results appeared to be a crucial point in the action cycle, where trust is most easily threatened. Trust appeared to be retained through dialogue, but their reaction to the written report (although there were few changes before it went out for all staff to read) forewarned me of possible difficulties ahead when it came to embracing change. To have set up a 'communicative space' (Kemmis, 2001) as part of the management of the study, where care staff and management could speak together about end-of-life care, might have facilitated greater responsibility and ownership for the study on the part of the NH and at the same time defuse the issue of insider/outsider.

Whether it was because I had learnt from my experience in NH1 about the need for greater regular dialogue with management, or that the staff I was working with in NH2 were more open to change and felt less threatened generally, or that I was slightly more removed from 'top' management was difficult to say. However, it was noticeable that the management and nurse manager at NH2 valued the importance of change and were particularly interested in developing end-of-life care. The written report was seen as constructive and there was eagerness to set up a multi-disciplinary group when it came to develop the adapted LCP which acted as a very convenient 'communicative space'.

Issues of power, authority, and change

Power needs to be shared between the researcher and those involved in the action research in order to learn from one another. Staff in both NH1 and NH2 were feeling more supported and empowered with their increasing knowledge of end of life care as a result of the actions (see Box 2.1). I was openly acknowledging how much I was learning from the staff. However, despite an eagerness by the management in NH1 to be part of the study at the beginning, I was realizing subtle changes in their attitude towards the project. The staff had also noticed, as reported in this evaluation feedback: '[The project] was welcomed enthusiastically initially by management and staff but the management soon lost interest and the support was not forthcoming from them to implement changes which would benefit caring the dying in this NH'. (N3, evaluation questionnaire, NH1) (Hockley, 2006). The nurse manager had attended the RdBGs but I had naively accepted the nurse manager's excuse of busyness as a legitimate reason for cancelling our monthly meetings together. I had reasoned to myself at the time that it did not matter since we seemed to be getting on well. However, without these regular meetings I had lost the opportunity to share concerns and my increasing rapport with the staff perhaps made her feel threatened.

Alongside this, management of NH1 felt that greater openness about death and dying might do more harm than good. However, the staff through the RdBGs had found a good way to support and develop their understanding about death and dying, but there was a need for more support from the management. Three staff had shared with me their reasons for handing in their notice but these were not the reasons given to management. Some further staff had mentioned to me that they were unhappy and were thinking of leaving. They wanted to feel more valued for the work they did. I wanted to draw management's attention to the matter because these staff were very committed to caring for older people in the nursing home. An opportunity arose after one of the RdBGs when the nurse manager and I were in the office. She had just told me about another staff member leaving. As the nurse manager and I sat in the office together, I posed the question as to why she felt staff might be leaving. We talked together about the need for staff to feel supported especially when residents were so frail. Unfortunately, my concern was misconstrued and the nurse manager reported me to the owners of the nursing home.

One of the owners suggested that I might be a threat to the nurse manager; however, I had seen the owners and nurse manager as all-powerful and very much in charge. The experience of the situation described above was a salutary lesson in maintaining a 'communicative space' when undertaking action research. I had been reading a non-academic book that threw light on issues to do with power and bringing about change. It described the difference between 'authority' and 'power'—the difference between having the right to do something (authority) and, having the ability to do something (power) (Cole, 2003). As I reflected I realized that the nurse manager had the authority but my ability/skill in palliative care had likely undermined that authority. When authority for whatever reason is weak in an organization, not recognizing the power of 'expert skill' in an area where staff are looking to be re-skilled is very dangerous. 'To have authority without power is degrading. To have power without authority is dangerous' (Cole, 2003: 14). Maybe my expert skill in palliative care unintentionally undermined her authority in the team.

Interpreting actions to build a model for the development of end-of-life care in nursing homes

One of the key features of critical action research is its ability both to develop practice, and at the same time contribute to a greater understanding of the subject being researched—in this case the development of end of life care for frail older people in nursing homes.

This study uncovered differences in caring for frail older people dying in nursing homes with those dying in mid-life (Hockley, 2002). For example, nursing home residents, an increasing number of whom have several different pathologies including advanced dementia, are cared for by staff, the majority of whom have little or no training, even though residents could be described as having advanced, progressive, non-curable disease (Doyle *et al.*, 1993: 3). In contrast, specialist palliative care/ hospice units are organized through a multi-disciplinary model of care that includes doctors, nurses, care assistants, pharmacists, physiotherapists, occupational therapists, and ward administrators.

As I reflected further, and re-read critical theorist Habermas (1987a; b), I realized that the actions that we had introduced in the NHs could in some manner correspond to Habermas's ideas around 'system' and 'lifeworld'. The LCP had become the necessary structure ('system') in the care of residents and their families before the death and the reflective de-briefing groups (RdBGs) that occurred after the death had highlighted the importance of the human component of staff ('lifeworld') in NHs. Here was the beginning of a model for development of end-of-life care in nursing homes that had arisen out of the action research study (see Figure 2.1). The model highlights this equal importance of the system and lifeworld.

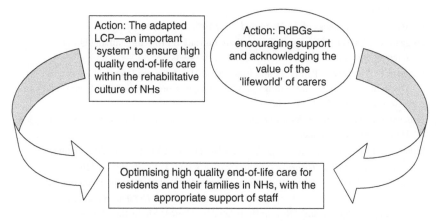

Fig. 2.1 The equal importance of 'lifeworld' and 'system' in the development of end-of-life care in nursing homes.

Conclusion

This chapter has highlighted aspects of using a critical theoretic approach to action research. It has briefly outlined critical social theory and emphasized the importance of reflexivity and praxis within such an approach to action research. A critical action research study carried out over a five-year period highlighted the importance of a participatory approach and the creation of a 'communicative space' which when present enables a greater democratic approach to change. Finally, the chapter highlighted a model to help with the development of high quality end-of-life care in nursing homes which was inductively derived from the process of undertaking this critical action research study.

References

Alvesson, M. and Skoldberg, K. (2000) *Reflexive Methodology: New Vistas for Qualitative Research*. London: Sage Publications Ltd.

Bellman, L. (1996) Changing Nursing Practice through Reflection on the Roper, Logan and Tierney Model: The Enhancement Approach to Action Research. *Journal of Advanced Nursing*, **24**: 129–38.

Bellman, L. (1999) *Nurse-led Change and Development*. PhD thesis. Steinberg Collection, Royal College of Nursing, London.

Carr, W. and Kemmis, S. (1986) *Becoming Critical: Education, Knowledge and Action Research*. London: The Falmer Press.

Cole, J. (2003) *Developing a Healing Ministry: A Training Manual for Churches*. London: New Wine.

Doyle, D., Hanks, G., and MacDonald, N. (1993) Introduction. In D. Doyle, G. Hanks, and N. MacDonald (eds), *Oxford Textbook of Palliative Medicine*, pp. 3–8. Oxford: Oxford Medical Publications.

Ellershaw, J. and Wilkinson, S. (2003) *Care of the Dying: A Pathway to Excellence*. Oxford: Oxford University Press.

Freire, P. (1970) *Pedagogy of the Oppressed*. New York: Seabury Press.

Froggatt, K. (2000) Evaluating a Palliative Care Education Project in Nursing Homes. *International Journal of Palliative Nursing*, **6**(3): 140–6.

Froggatt, K., Hockley, J., Parker, D. and Brazil, K. (2011) A System Lifeworld Perspective on Dying in Long Term Care Settings for Older People: Contested States in Contested Places. *Health and Place*, **17**(1): 263–8.

Habermas, J. (1972) *Knowledge and Human Interest* (translated by Jeremy J. Shapiro). London: Heinemann Educational.

Habermas, J. (1974) *Theory and Practice* (translated by John Viertal). London: Heinemann.

Habermas, J. (1984) *The Theory of Communicative Action. Vol. I: Reason and the Rationalization of Society* (translated by Thomas McCarthy). London: Heinemann.

Habermas, J. (1987) *The Theory of Communicative Action. Vol. II: Lifeworld and System: A Critique of Functionalist Reason* (translated by Thomas McCarthy). Polity Press: Cambridge.

Held D. (1980) *Introduction to Critical Theory: Horkheimer to Habermas*. Polity Press: Cambridge.

Hockley, J. (2002) Organizational Structures for Enhancing Standards of Palliative Care. In: J. Hockley and D. Clark (eds), *Palliative Care for Older People in Care Homes*, pp. 165–81. Buckingham: Open University Press.

Hockley, J. (2006) Developing High Quality End of Life Care in Nursing Care Homes: An Action Research Study. Unpublished PhD thesis, University of Edinburgh.

Hockley, J. and Froggatt, K. (2006) The Development of Palliative Care Knowledge in Care Homes for Older People: The Place of Action Research. *Palliative Medicine*, **20**(8): 835–43.

Holter, I. and Schwartz-Barcott, D. (1993) Action Research: What is it? How Has it Been Used and How Can it be Used in Nursing? *Journal of Advanced Nursing*, **18**: 298–304.

Kemmis, S. (1985) Action Research and the Politics of Reflection. In: D. Boud, R. Keogh, and D. Walker (eds), *Reflection: Turning Experience into Learning*, pp. 139–63. London: Kogan Page.

Kemmis, S. (2001) Exploring the Relevance of Critical Theory for Action Research: Emancipatory Action Research in the Footsteps of Jurgen Habermas. In: P. Reason and H. Bradbury (eds), *Handbook of Action Research: Participator Inquiry and Practice*, pp. 91–102. London: Sage Publications.

Kemmis, S. and McTaggart, R. (1988) *The Action Research Planner*. Deakin: Deakin University Press.

Kincheloe, J.L. and McLaren, P.L. (1994) Rethinking Critical Theory and Qualitative Research. In: N.K. Denzin, and Y.S. Lincoln (eds), *Handbook of Qualitative Research*, pp. 138–57. London: Sage Publications.

Manley, K. (2000) Organisational Culture and Consultant Nurse Outcomes: Part 1 Organisational Culture. *Nursing Standard*, **30**(14): 34–8.

Manley, K. (2001) Consultant Nurse: Concept, Processes, Outcomes. Unpublished doctoral thesis. London: University of Manchester/RCN Institute.

Marx, K. (1845) *Theses on Feuerbach XI. Marx/Engel Internet Archive*. Available at http://www.marxists.org/archive/marx/works/1845/theses/theses.htm (accessed December 2005).

Meyer, J. (1995) Lay Participation in Care in a Hospital Setting: An Action Research Study. Unpublished PhD thesis, King's College London, University of London.

Meyer, J. (2000) Using Qualitative Methods in Health Related Action Research. *British Medical Journal*, **320**: 178–81.

Meyer, J. and Batehup, L. (1997) Action Research in Healthcare Practice: Nature, Present Concerns and Future Possibilities. *NTresearch*, **2**(3): 175–84.

Nolan, M. and Grant, G. (1993) Action Research and Quality of Care: A Mechanism for Agreeing Basic Values as A Precursor to Change. *Journal of Advanced Nursing*, **18**: 305–11.

Rafferty, A. M., Allcock, N., and Lathlean, J. (1996) The Theory/Practice 'Gap': Taking Issue With the Issue. *Journal of Advanced Nursing*, **23**(4): 685–91.

Rolfe, G. (1993) Closing the Theory-Practice Gap: A Model of Nursing Praxis. *Journal of Clinical Nursing*, **2**: 173–7.

Rolfe, G. (1997) Nursing Praxis: A Zealot Responds. *Journal of Advanced Nursing*, **25**: 426–7.

Rolfe, G., Freshwater, D., and Jasper, M. (2001) *Critical Reflection for Nursing and the Helping Professions: A User's Guide*. London: Palgrave Macmillan.

Stringer, E.T. (1996) *Action Research: A Handbook for Practitioners*. Thousand Oaks, CA: Sage Publications.

Titchen, A. (2000) *Professional Craft Knowledge in Patient-centred Nursing and the Facilitation of its Development*. PhD thesis. Oxford: Ashdale Press.

Titchen, A. and Binnie, A. (1993) Research partnerships: Collaborative Action Research in Nursing. *Journal of Advanced Nursing*, **18**(6): 858–65.

Webb, G. (1996) Becoming Critical of Action Research for Development. In: O. Zuber-Skerritt (ed.), *New Directions in Action Research*, pp. 137–61. London: RoutledgeFalmer.

Williamson G.R., Bellman, L., and Webster J. (eds) (2012) *Action Research in Nursing and Healthcare*. Los Angeles: Sage.

Chapter 3

Organizational and health system change through participatory research

Katharina Heimerl and Klaus Wegleitner

Dignified persons require dignified organizations

In this chapter we want to focus on organization rather than on individuals. We do not do so because we think that people do not matter; neither do we think that organization and person are exclusionary concepts. On the contrary, it is our conviction, that the respect for the person (Kitwood, 1997) also includes organizational conditions and structures that value the people who are doing the caring along with those being cared for in organizations (Brooker, 2006). Frail and vulnerable individuals, as in palliative care, need and deserve dignified and respectful organizations. Therefore, for us neglecting the important role that organizations and their structures play in providing palliative care means denying adequate care for those most concerned, for the 'patients and their families facing the problems associated with life-threatening illness' (WHO, 2002: 83).

It is our experience that organizational structures often leave those who are involved in palliative care with a feeling of powerlessness. Sentences such as: 'There is nothing I can do about it' come to their minds. For many, the solution seems to be to undergo more palliative care training, often with a special emphasis on attitudes in palliative care. Nevertheless, we believe that even the best trained persons with the most authentic attitude in palliative care cannot compensate for the deficits of low-quality organizations.

In this chapter we want to convey to the readers that there is much that can be done to change organizations and their cultures and structures, provided there is: first, a common effort; second, the willingness to look closely at organizations, their cultures and structures; and finally, systematic and sustainable measures to change the culture. Action research will be introduced as a very helpful tool to foster this kind of social change.

This chapter considers the place of organizations in palliative care provision, organizations as complex social systems, the place of action research as an approach to change the palliative care culture in and between organizations, and, finally, we present a case study illustrating these elements in practice.

The place of organizations in palliative care delivery

The WHO aims to develop and establish palliative care as a worldwide care available for terminally ill people and their families, independent of their social, economical, and ethnic background (WHO, 2002). In addition to medical challenges, the major barriers in end-of-life care consist of socio-economic, cultural, and ethical problems (Stjernswärd and Clark, 2004). Introducing a palliative care culture within society requires a public health and health promotion approach (Kellehear, 1999; 2008; Stjernswärd, 2007). The key challenge for improving end-of-life care is to establish a dignified culture of dying within organizations (Heller, 1996). Developing a palliative care culture cannot be restricted to processes within organizations, but almost always requires communication between organizations as well as social integration at a community level, as will be shown later.

Modern societies have created organizations to deal with the challenges they are confronted with. Public goods are increasingly processed and handled in and by organizations, such as education in schools, research in universities, health in hospitals, or care needs in nursing homes. In other words modern society is a 'society of organizations' (Etzioni, 1967):

> Our society is an organizational society. We are born in organizations, educated by organizations and most of us spend most of our lives working for organizations. We spend much of our leisure time paying, playing and praying in organizations. Most of us will die in an organization and when the time comes for burial, the largest organization of all—the state—must grant official permission.
>
> (Etzioni, 1967: 1)

In industrialized countries people do not only live in organizations, they also die in organizations, and this is a message that pervades the entire book. In many countries up to 80% of the population die in institutions such as hospitals, care homes, or nursing homes (e.g. Jaspers and Schindler, 2004). There exists a well known paradox in palliative care: up to 80% of the population say they do not want to die in an institution; they want to die at home. A recent European Study concludes that between 56% (Portugal) and 83% (the Netherlands) of the population wish to die at home (Gomes *et al.*, 2012).

From the very beginning the relationship between the hospice movement/palliative care and organizations has been both critical and developmental. Both founders of the modern hospice movement, Elisabeth Kübler-Ross and Dame Cicely Saunders, maintained a very critical attitude towards the hospital. Cicely Saunders founded her own organization to care for the dying—St Christopher's Hospice in London. This was the birth of a type of organization that is now called specialist palliative care (as opposed to generalist palliative care), and exists today in a wide range of organizations, such as hospices, palliative care units, specialist palliative care teams, and hospice teams. Only a very small percentage of the population has access to specialist palliative care services, despite the increase in demand. In Germany it is estimated that only between 3–5% of the dying patients are cared for in specialist palliative care services (Jaspers and Schindler, 2004).

The relationship between hospice movement and palliative care with respect to organizations can be characterized as fugitive. The early hospice movement attempted to escape from organizations; a dynamic that persists in some aspects even today. Up until recently the hospice movement was confronted with the need to balance the original ideas of the civil movement on one hand and at the same time to strive to develop 'palliative care for all' as summarized by Twycross: 'However, at the end of the day, if we are truly to honour Cicely Saunders, palliative care must remain a movement with momentum, combining creative charisma with inevitable bureaucratic routinization' (Twycross, 2008: 7).

Organizations as complex social systems

McNiff defines organizations as 'contexts in which people come together for a variety of reasons to achieve commonly agreed goals' (McNiff, 2000: 55). Whilst we agree with this definition we introduce our understanding of organizational change processes based primarily on German system theory (Luhmann, 1984; 2006; Willke, 1995; 1996; 2005). Organizations can be understood as complex social systems, which steadily pursue a goal and exhibit a formal structure. Ideally, the activities of organizational members should be concentrated on a common mission or goal (Kieser and Walgenbach, 2003), a similar precept to that identified by McNiff (2000).

According to German system theory, an organization consists of communication not of people (Luhmann, 1984). Men and women as physical members of an organization are considered to be 'environment'; however, their communications and decisions form the substance of organizations.

In a similar way to systems theory, McNiff states: 'The subject matter of organization studies still remains the organization itself as an object, rather than people within organizational contexts' (McNiff, 2000: 55). Furthermore, organizations are considered to be 'autopoetic': they are reproducing and re-creating themselves in a continuing process. External stimuli (such as action research projects) are selected, perceived, and processed in ways that are unpredictable for others. The organization decides what is relevant for its development and self-reproduction. This implies that there is a permanent need to make decisions in organizations. The focus in organizations, according to Luhmann (2006), lies on decisions. Organizational development can offer knowledge for orientation as well as methods for self-reflection and self-description (Willke, 1995).

We think that this is also true for action research. The goal is to establish 'reflective loops' that help organizations to observe and describe themselves and to generate decisions (Luhmann, 2006). By providing reflective loops action research helps to create spaces where organizations can deal with their problems by changing routine processes and standard procedures. For example, a workshop in a nursing home that involves different professions and hierarchies, and starts with the question: 'How can we respond adequately to the needs of our residents?' or: 'How are we dealing with death, dying and bereavement in our nursing home?' provides such a reflective space that interrupts routine and offers a chance for innovative decisions (Heimerl, 2008).

Action research as an intervention to develop palliative care provision in and between organizations

The palliative care concept as published by the World Health Organization (WHO, 2002) is an expression of explicit norms and values. Projects that aim at integrating palliative care in organizations at the same time try to alter the basic values in organizations by introducing the values held by palliative care. Edgar Schein's concept of organizational culture provides a very helpful framework for understanding the dynamics created by projects that aim at implementing palliative care.

Schein's concept relies on the following definition of organizational culture: 'A pattern of basic assumptions—invented, discovered, or developed by a given group as it learns to cope with its problems of external adaptation and internal integration—that has worked well enough to be considered valid and, therefore to be taught to new members as the correct way to perceive, think, and feel in relation to those problems' (Schein, 1987: 9).

Schein stresses the fact that organizational culture is not something an organization *has*, rather it *is* organizational culture. He distinguishes three levels of organizational culture:

1. Artefacts—visible or audible behaviour patterns which are often difficult or even impossible to decipher.

2. Espoused values—the sense of what 'ought to be' as distinct from what is. Such values remain conscious and are explicitly articulated; they serve the normative and moral function of guiding members of the group in how to deal with certain key situations.

3. Basic underlying assumptions—implicit and unconscious assumptions, and therefore cannot be confronted, but at the same time are non-debatable. They shape the communication cultures in organizations and give the organization its unique characteristics (Schein, 1987: 14ff.).

Organizational culture can only be changed when there are times and settings for reflection and collective learning that help to understand and challenge the basic underlying assumptions.

The ideas of system theory have been integrated into action research work. Burns (2007) has coined the notion of 'systemic action research'. He points out that the term 'systemic action research' has been used by other authors before. Although the focus of these authors is diverse, they share a concern to take into account the wider context within which issues are situated (Burns, 2007: 10). Burns refers to Anglo-American systems theory and applies system thinking to practice. In his book he describes systems as: 'Constructions that enable us to see the different factors that are important, the connections between them, and the boundaries around them' (Burns, 2007: 7). Systemic action research: 'Combines inquiry with action as a means of stimulating and supporting change and as a way of assessing the impact of that change' (Burns, 2007: 11). It 'is a process through which communities and organizations can adapt and respond purposefully to their constantly changing environments' (Burns, 2007: 1).

Burns (2007) is very clear about the fact that change in organizations is 'non-linear' and that it is not possible to predict what effect a certain external intervention will generate within the organization:

> Social and economic problems are highly complex and affected by multiple factors. When these factors combine they do not produce predictable outcomes. To understand the dynamics of change we have to look at them in their context and find ways of making visible some of the systemic connections that affect them. This opens up the possibility for interventions that shift outcomes in the direction that we desire. We can never predict

the detailed outcomes but we can make judgments about the direction of travel when we can see more of the picture. Despite this, things will not happen as we expect, so we need a process that allows us to change course flexibly and quickly.

(Burns, 2007: 39)

There is a narrow boundary between action research and organizational development (OD) (Frohman *et al.*, 1982). Both approaches refer to Kurt Lewin as a common founder and they both 'recognize that any action with respect to a client system is an intervention and may have some effect on the client system' (Frohman *et al.*, 1982: 199). The most important difference is that action research not only brings about change but also adds to new behavioural scientific knowledge. Argyris *et al.* (1985) in their 'action science' approach to organizational development also emphasize that action science aims at 'advancing basic knowledge, while also solving practical problems' (see Chapter 5).

Hospice and Palliative Care Plan in Tyrol, Austria: a case study of participatory research in organizations and healthcare systems

In the Austrian province Tyrol a three-year, multi-level organizational action research project was undertaken with the following objectives:

♦ To develop a regional specific concept for integrated palliative care.

♦ To generate knowledge and foster communication among local actors and stakeholders.

♦ To integrate palliative care into the regional healthcare systems.

♦ To supervise the integration-processes and consult local healthcare policy.

The project was commissioned by the Tyrolean Health Fund, a funding agency that consists of representatives of social insurance and of health and social government on a provincial level. The project was laid out in three phases that each lasted a year: needs assessment, planning of measures, and implementing measures. The integration of palliative care focused on two remote model regions (Lienz and Reutte) in the province.

Participation and involvement of local stakeholders in this regional palliative care development process were undertaken at different levels as shown in Figure 3.1.

Attention was given to three types of intervention: development of palliative culture in primary care organizations; development and acceptance of specialist palliative care structures; and integration and governance of the hospice and palliative care plan in Tyrol (see Figure 3.1).

Participation was encouraged through collective data collection, needs assessment, and evaluation on a regional (model region) as well as on a supra-regional (province of Tyrol) level (see Figure 3.2).

The following project structure was established:

A. Organizational level

The action research project offered possibilities to further develop organizational palliative culture processes within different care settings. Workshops and task

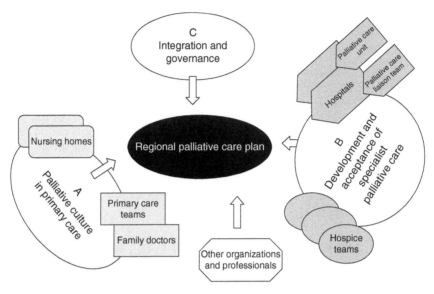

Fig. 3.1 Architecture of the project: project partners and levels of intervention.

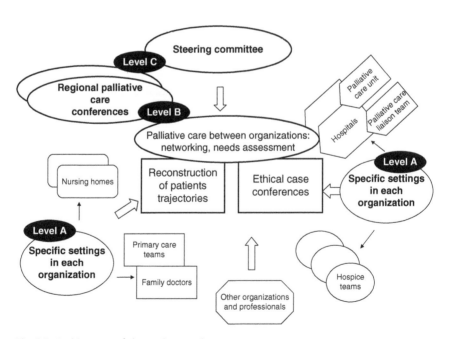

Fig. 3.2 Architecture of the project: project structures.

forces were held for palliative care in two hospitals and in three nursing homes of the model regions. A palliative care course was established that offered continuing education for all stakeholders in and beyond all involved organizations. The project process also served to develop and establish structures of specialized palliative care services and units, specifically for the two model regions. To foster the acceptance of these new structures in the in-patient area as well as in the home care setting was a major challenge.

B. Inter-organizational level

A platform was initiated, where members of all involved organizations and voluntary hospice groups could participate. This has enabled the stakeholders to develop a perspective of an adequate regional palliative care culture. As an example, one methodical tool, the 'reconstruction of patient trajectories' is discussed in more detail below. The participating actors developed plans for necessary measures and steps to further the implementation of palliative care in the model regions. At this level during the assessment phase, considerable and sustainable participation was generated, and networking processes were started. The processes yielded high expectations of the involved actors regarding sustainable financing of the planned measures.

C. Policy and management level

At a province level a steering committee was established that brought together all representatives of the commissioning agency. Furthermore a regional palliative care conference was established in each of the two model regions. In all three structures common goals and interests were discussed, strategic decisions and conceptual suggestions were debated. Considerable power was exercised by the actors in the model regions who were involved in planning specific measures to implement palliative care. This resulted in extensive negotiations between the model regions and the funding body mediated by the researchers and the project managing team. Finally almost all planned measures could be implemented.

Reconstructing patients' trajectories—an example of participatory research at an inter-organizational level

A major challenge in implementing palliative care is that patients' trajectories at the end of their lives occur across different organizations not alongside. There is a lack of good communication and cooperation at the intersection between these different organizations. In our project, we invited representatives of different professions (doctors, nurses, social workers) and healthcare organizations (hospital, home care, care and nursing homes) to participate in several workshops to analyse the trajectories of collectively cared for patients after their death. We asked the question: 'What was the patient's trajectory in the last six months of her/his life?' The data were collected with the help of a structured questionnaire and through group discussions. The workshop participants retrospectively identified the places of care of selected and collectively cared for patients. They then analysed care interfaces, challenges in regional end-of-life care, shared their experiences, exchanged know how and developed prospects of advancing palliative care in the model region, in and across the healthcare organizations. Among the major results of the process was the insight that to reconstruct the entire trajectory of the last six months of a patient requires a joint effort. None of the health professionals could do it by her/himself. The insights of the workshops were used as departure points for developing measures to improve cooperation in palliative care in the model regions.

Key elements of participatory research in organizational and regional palliative care processes

Based on our experiences with projects that aim at developing palliative care culture within and in between organizations, we have identified the following key elements for participatory research in palliative care.

Participation and democracy

In order to encourage developmental potential, all people concerned should be engaged in project development. Healthcare planning and developing organizational palliative care culture must be based on a democratic process, that is, including patients, professionals, and spokespersons on an equal basis with regards to care options (Beresford and Cross, 2011). One main indicator for a sustainable development of palliative culture in organizations is the shift from a hierarchical style of leading to a participatory style of leading. It is important to highlight that participation is not easy for patients at the end of life whose strength is decreasing as death approaches. However, in the same way as autonomy, participation for palliative care patients can be realized with the help of relationships. It may therefore be appropriate to speak about 'relational participation' in palliative care.

Empowerment

Sustainable changes should be introduced through self-development rather than through imposed, one-sided intervention by external consultants. Action research should aim at handing over co-ownership of the project to all people involved in the study. Empowerment is described as one of the key aspects of community based participatory research (CBPR) (Minkler and Wallerstein, 2002). In Wallersteins' words, empowerment is 'a social action process by which individuals, communities and organizations gain mastery over their lives in the context of changing their social and political environment to improve equity and quality of life' (Wallerstein, 1992: 198).

A distinction has to be made between 'empowering' organizations, which means that the organization provides opportunities for people to gain control over their lives; and, 'empowered' organizations, which are capable of influencing policy decisions, of creating alternative services, and of networking with other organizations (Zimmermann quoted in Minkler et al., 2001).

Appreciative organizational diagnosis

The first phase of a participatory research project in palliative care is of particular importance. In this phase the status quo of the provision of palliative care in an organization is assessed. Usually there is a lot of experience in all healthcare organizations with provision of care for dying patients. This experience has to be respected and valued in action research projects. If the project succeeds to establish an appreciative process of self reflection by the major stakeholders, implementation of palliative care has already started. Stakeholders in organizations that analyse their own practice and ask themselves such questions as: 'In what ways have we been successful in caring for chronically ill and dying patients in our organization?' or 'What are our potentials for developing the care for chronically ill and dying patients?' generate an enormous power (in the sense of em-*power*-ment) to change their own routines and to develop the care they are giving to their patients (see Chapter 6).

If this phase of 'organizational diagnosis' is successful in generating relevant knowledge as well as linking the stakeholders with each other, this constitutes a solid ground for sustainability of change. The more perspectives and levels of the organization—or of the healthcare system—are included in the intervention, the more the palliative care process is sustainable.

Complex problems require complex solutions

The right balance between the necessary reduction of complexity and at the same time adequate complexity has to be found in organizations in order to enable good decision making processes. Whether a problem can be solved adequately by an organization depends on the right degree of complexity—because organizations 'can only respond to complexity by complexity' (Baecker, 1999: 27ff.). In other words, complex problems require complex solutions. 'A holistic approach to intervention is crucial because complex issues cannot be adequately comprehended in isolation from the wider system of which they are a part' (Burns, 2007: 1).

In our work in bringing about change in palliative care organizations, we have found it very helpful to handle complexity in action research projects by integrating the perspectives of the relevant actors or stakeholders (see Figure 3.3).

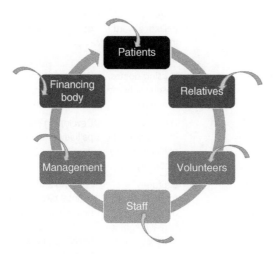

Fig. 3.3 Importance of different stakeholders' perspectives in participatory research in organizations.

Inter-disciplinary and multiple perspectives

Patient needs and their symptoms are multifaceted at the end of life. Palliative care therefore has to be an interdisciplinary concept. All professions involved in the care process depend on each other in facing care challenges. Due to their complexity, viable and innovative corrections to care problems cannot be tackled by focusing only on professional and field-specific perspectives. The most potential for development and learning lies in 'astonishing links' ('überraschende Vernetzungen', Grossmann and Scala, 1994: 98), that means connecting perspectives that have not been linked before (e.g. the perspective of housekeepers with the perspective of nurses in nursing homes). This helps to question and alter routines.

Different interventions at different levels

In action research projects that aim at fostering change *between* organizations—what Burns calls 'large scale organizational action research' (Burns, 2007)—there is a need for intervention on different levels. On each level different dynamics of self-organization and intervention occur. Willke (2005: 52) states that: 'A prerequisite [for successful intervention] is the insight, that there are completely different levels to construct a system' (see Table 3.1).

Table 3.1 Levels to construct a system in palliative care (based on Willke 2005: 53)

Level	Characteristics of communication	Examples in palliative care	Possible action research interventions
Individual/ person	Direct	Older person, guest in hospice, palliative care nurse, manager	Research guided need assessment by staff
Group	Informal	Team of palliative ward in hospital, care giving family	Evaluation, feedback, and discussion of needs assessment
Organization	Formal	Nursing homes, hospitals, home care teams	Developing communication structures, implementing case and care management
Subsystem in society	Formal	Dementia care in a community, palliative care in a country	Developing community based palliative care and solidarity-networks
Society	Media civil society movements	Attitudes towards dying, death, and bereavement in society	Enabling and encouraging the societal discourse about dying, death, bereavement; solidarity and social justice in society through a public health, participatory action research project

Data from Willke, H., *Systemtheorie II, Interventionstheorie: Grundzüge einer Theorie der Intervention in komplexe Systeme*, Fourth Edition, UTB, Stuttgart, Germany, Copyright © 2005.

Inter-organization

Palliative care is not limited to the inner-organizational procedure of dealing with dying, death, and grief. Proper care at the end of a life must be organized across organizations. It therefore is essential to incorporate all care institutions when developing a regional palliative culture. The willingness to cooperate has to be fostered. The basis consists of a common and coordinated palliative care approach by the regional organizations and care systems. Collective learning, and cognitive production processes function as the premise for organizational and regional development in palliative care.

Relationship between individual and organizational learning processes

Palliative care development processes require the interaction between individual development and organizational learning. Learning organizations need to arrange continuous settings of collective reflection, dealing with questions of palliative care culture, in which as many staff members as possible are involved. Managing organizational learning means dealing with complex and nonlinear processes. Within the scope of action research projects, the organization of reflective contexts and 'reflective architectures' (Zepke, 2005) is encouraging the correlation between individual and organizational learning processes.

Relationship between theory and practice

Palliative care concepts can neither be planned by the scientific community alone, nor are they based solely on the experiences of palliative caregivers. Strategies for integration in palliative care evolve from an exchange between theory and practice. Developmental processes in palliative care bring together a wealth of knowledge from professionals, various disciplines, from players in the healthcare system, and, most important, from persons concerned.

Cultural sensitivity reflecting regional characteristics

The needs and wishes of those concerned, and the structures of a specific health care system, have grown out of, and are strongly tied to, their regional and cultural context. Implementing palliative care is a process that must respect cultural distinctions and values, and the different ways in which organizational systems work; not one-sided political planning of palliative care services, but a cooperative, communal shaping of cultural spaces for living and dying must be placed to the forefront (Conway, 2011).

Conclusion

Frail and vulnerable people at the end of their lives deserve dignified and respectful organizations. If we neglect the importance that organizations and their structures play in palliative care, we are in danger of denying adequate care to those who are most in need at the end of life.

To this end, we have found participatory research to be very powerful in fostering social change in organizations and in establishing community based palliative care cultures. Key issues within participatory action research are participation, democratization, interdisciplinary and multi-perspective knowledge development, and self-development—that is, empowerment. However, organizations are complex, and successful implementation of palliative care requires a change in established communication and decision-making structures. The basis for a sustainable development of palliative care culture consists of a collective and coordinated approach by the regional organizations as well as the social and healthcare systems.

Implementation of palliative care in healthcare systems can only succeed by developing organizations, their subsystems and their local structural environments. Of particular importance is an awareness of cultural and regional distinctions and a broad participation among local players: the healthcare professionals and the people concerned—the patients and their relatives.

The key challenge of palliative care is not simply to change and develop the ways care is provided. Social relationship patterns and solidarities must be strengthened and locally applied to the formal organizational structure of care provision. Organic, regional, self-development processes in palliative care can be fostered through participatory research processes.

References

Argyris, C., Putnam, R., and Smith McLain, D. (1985) *Action Science*. San Francisco, London: Jossey-Bass.

Baecker, D. (1999) *Organisation als System. Aufsätze*. Frankfurt am Main: Suhrkamp.

Beresford, P. and Cross, S. (2011) Involvement and Empowerment at the End of Life: Overcoming the Barriers. In: S. Conway (ed.), *Governing Death and Loss: Empowerment, Involvement and Participation*, pp. 53–62. Oxford: Oxford University Press.

Brooker, D. (2006) *Person Centred Dementia Care: Making Services Better*. London, Philadelphia: Jessica Kingsley Publishers.

Burns, D. (2007) *Systemic Action Research: A Strategy for Whole System Change*. Bristol, UK: The Policy Press.

Conway, S. (2011) *Governing Death and Loss. Empowerment, Involvement and Participation*. Oxford: Oxford University Press.

Etzioni, A. (1967) *Modern Organizations*. Englewood Cliffs. New Jersey: Prentice Hall.

Frohman, M., Sashkin, M., and Kavanagh, M. (1982) Action-research as Applied to Organization Development. In: M. Plovnik., R. Fry, and W. Burke (eds), *Organization Development: Exercises, Cases and Readings*, pp. 197–209. Boston, Toronto: Little, Brown and Company.

Gomes, B., Higginson, I.J., Calanzani, N., *et al.* (on behalf of PRISMA) (2012) Preferences for Place of Death if Faced with Advanced Cancer: A Population Survey in England, Flanders, Germany, Italy, the Netherlands, Portugal and Spain. *Annals of Oncology*, published online 16 February 2012.

Grossmann, R., and Scala, K. (1994) *Gesundheit durch Projekte fördern*. München: Juventa, Weinheim.

Heimerl, K. (2008) *Orte zum Leben—Orte zum Sterben: Palliative Care in Organisationen umsetzen*. Freiburg im Breisgau: Lambertus.

Heller, A. (1996) Sterben in Organisationen. In: R. Grossmann (ed.) *Gesundheitsförderung und Public Health, Öffentliche Gesundheit durch Organisation entwickeln*, pp. 214–31. Wien: Facultas.

Jaspers, B. and Schindler, T. (2004) *Stand der Palliativmedizin und Hospizarbeit in Deutschland im Vergleich zu ausgewählten Staaten (Belgien, Frankreich, Großbritannien, Niederlande, Norwegen, Österreich, Polen, Schweden, Schweiz, Spanien).* Auftraggeber: Enquete-Kommission des Bundestages 'Ethik und Recht der modernen Medizin'. Available at http://www.lönsapo.de/öpag-nds/dokument/gutachten-palliativ-brd.pdf (accessed 18 March 2012).

Kellehear, A. (1999) *Health Promoting Palliative Care.* Oxford: Oxford University Press.

Kellehear, A. (2008) Health Promotion and Palliative Care. In: G. Mitchell (ed.), *Palliative Care, a Patient-centred Approach*, pp. 139–56. Oxford: Radcliff Publishing.

Kieser, A. and Walgenbach, P. (2003) *Organisation.* Stuttgart: Schäffer Poeschel.

Kitwood T. (1997) *Dementia Reconsidered: The Person Comes First.* Buckingham, UK: Open University Press.

Luhmann, N. (1984) *Soziale Systeme: Grundriss einer allgemeinen Theorie.* Frankfurt am Main: Suhrkamp.

Luhmann, N. (2006) *Organisation und Entscheidung*, 2nd edn. Wiesbaden: VS Verlag für Sozialwissenschaften.

McNiff, J. (2000) *Action Research in Organisations.* London, New York: Rutledge.

Minkler, M., Thompson, M., Bell, J., and Rose, K. (2001) Contributions of Community Involvement to Organizational-Level Empowerment: The Federal Healthy Start Experience. *Health Education & Behavior*, **28**(6): 783–807.

Minkler, M. and Wallerstein, N. (2002) *Community-Based Participatory Research for Health.* San Francisco, London: Jossey-Bass.

Schein, E.H. (1987) *Organizational Culture and Leadership.* San Francisco, London: Jossey-Bass.

Stjernswärd, J. (2007) Palliative Care: The Public Health Strategy. *Journal of Public Health Policy*, **28**(1): 42–55.

Stjernswärd, J. and Clark, D. (2004) Palliative Medicine: A Global Perspective. In: D. Doyle, G. Hanks, N. Cherny, and K. Calman (eds), *Oxford Textbook of Palliative Medicine*, 3rd edn, pp. 1199–222. Oxford: Oxford University Press.

Twycross, R. (2008) Patient Care: Past, Present, and Future. *Omega*, **56**(1): 7–19.

Wallerstein, N. (1992) Powerlessness, Empowerment and Health: Implications for Health Promotion Programs. *American Journal of Health Promotion*, **6**(3):197–205.

World Health Organization (2002) *National Cancer Control Programmes: Policies and Managerial Guidelines,* 2nd edn, pp. 83–4. Geneva: World Health Organization.

Willke, H. (1995) *Systemtheorie III: Steuerungstheorie.* Stuttgart, Jena: Fischer.

Willke, H. (1996) *Systemtheorie I: Grundlagen*, 5th edn. Stuttgart, Jena: Fischer.

Willke, H. (2005) *Systemtheorie II, Interventionstheorie: Grundzüge einer Theorie der Intervention in komplexe Systeme*, 4th edn. Stuttgart: UTB.

Zepke, G. (2005) *Reflexionsarchitekturen—Evaluierung als Beitrag zum Organisationslernen.* Heidelberg: Carl Auer.

Zimmerman M. (2000) Empowerment Theory: psychological, organizational and community levels of analysis. In: J. Rappaport and E. Seidman (eds), *Handbook of Community Psychology*, pp. 43–63. New York: Plenum.

Chapter 4

Capacity development in participatory action research

Mary Lou Kelley and Margaret McKee

Capacity development in long-term care homes through participatory action research

The purpose of this chapter is to propose and illustrate an integrative framework that can be used to guide participatory action research in order to develop palliative care programmes within long-term care (LTC) homes for elderly people. The framework consists of participatory action research (PAR) as an overarching approach, capacity development model, and four practice principles: cultural competence, empowerment, relational ethics, and partnerships (See Figure 4.1). Based on five years of experience conducting PAR with LTC homes in Ontario, Canada, the authors offer this framework as a resource to guide the work of other researchers and long-term care homes who wish to develop palliative care programmes. The authors have also used PAR to develop palliative care capacity in rural and First Nations communities, indicating that this approach has applicability beyond long-term care homes (Kelley *et al.*, 2011; Prince and Kelley, 2010).

Importance of palliative care research for long-term care homes

The urgency to provide palliative care services in LTC homes in Canada is growing because up to 90% of all residents now live in care homes right until death (Wowchuk *et al.*, 2007). Residents today have a high burden of chronic and terminal disease and high rates of Alzheimer's disease or related dementias (Wowchuk, 2006) that create care challenges due to communication, functional, and behavioural problems (Sachs *et al.*, 2004). Frequent causes of death are: pneumonia, coronary artery disease, congestive heart failure, cancer, and stroke (Reynolds *et al.*, 2002).

Given these characteristics, it is not surprising that almost fifty percent of residents die within the year in Ontario long-term care homes, with most residents dying within two years of their admission (Palliative Alliance, 2010). Common end-of-life symptoms, such as pain, incontinence, fatigue (Reynolds *et al.*, 2002), constipation (Casarett *et al.*, 2001), shortness of breath, restlessness, and agitation (Ley, 1989), indicate a need for palliative pain and symptom management. Dying residents would benefit from a palliative care approach that addresses not only physical symptoms but the

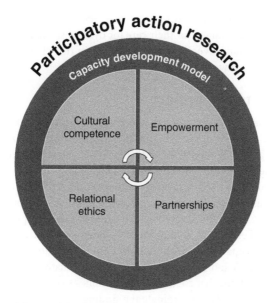

Fig. 4.1 Framework for participatory action research.

psychological, social, and spiritual issues at the end of life: issues of loss and grief, and practical end-of-life/death management concerns of residents and their families (Ferris *et al.*, 2002). Despite the need and benefits of palliative care for residents in long-term care, formalized palliative care programmes are rare in these settings.

Having a palliative care programme is currently not mandatory for LTC homes in Ontario and palliative care programmes do not have dedicated funding within long-term care homes (Ministry of Health and Long Term Care, 2007). This means that long-term care homes that wish to offer palliative care programmes must do so through developing capacity within their existing human and financial resources. Implementing the framework presented in this chapter offers long-term care homes a strategy to develop palliative care programmes using a process of capacity development.

Research has documented that organizational culture in LTC homes is a major barrier to the provision of palliative care (Foner, 1995). One aspect of current culture is that front-line unregistered care workers—called personal support workers (PSWs) in our province—who provide 80% of direct resident care, have minimal palliative care training and little input into resident care planning (QPC-LTC Alliance, 2010). The early findings of our research indicated that PSWs viewed giving care to dying people as an important part of their work which gave great meaning to their lives (QPC-LTC Alliance, 2010). They talked about the development of family-like bonds with residents and expressed their commitment to provide highly personalized care, especially at end of life (Sims-Gould *et al.*, 2010). At the same time, PSWs reported having problems communicating their perceptions of resident care needs with registered nursing staff and felt that they had little personal control or influence over their work (QPC-LTC Alliance, 2010). Over the past three years, using this framework and engaging PSWs in PAR has resulted in them feeling more confident in their competencies and more valued for their care for dying residents by other staff within the organization. Qualitative data presented later in this chapter illustrate PSWs' increased sense of empowerment.

Introduction to the project

The purpose of our five-year research, which commenced in 2009, was to improve quality of life for people who are dying in LTC by creating formalized palliative care programmes that can be sustained within the LTC home environment beyond completion of the project (see www.palliativealliance.ca).

Capacity development (Kelley, 2007) was chosen as the model for the research as we view LTC homes as relational and geographic communities. We adopted the Canadian Hospice Palliative Care model of care to guide our vision of a comprehensive palliative care programme (Ferris *et al.*, 2002). We developed an alliance of partnerships as resources for LTC capacity development, including four homes as study sites, 31 researchers with a wide range of methodological and palliative care expertise, and 43 community organizations that could assist LTC homes to deliver aspects of palliative care. Alliance members also disseminate the findings of the research to their stakeholder groups.

For our research, PAR was chosen as the overarching approach most appropriate to develop LTC capacity in palliative care. Participatory action research is an approach of action research that has an orientation towards action and change. A distinguishing issue is the degree to which the researcher maintains control of the research process. The degree of participant involvement varies on a continuum from: researchers consulting the community's views (least involvement); to designing the study and then collecting data with the help of the community; to the community working closely with researchers; to total participant control (most involvement) (Kemmis and McTaggart, 2000; 2005). Our research embraced the highest degree of participant involvement, with LTC staff becoming members of the research team and participating in all aspects of project decision making and execution. We chose PAR because research on capacity development has demonstrated that changes in organizational culture and practice are most sustainable when these changes are planned and executed by those most directly involved.

We will now describe the components of the framework we used for conducting this research and illustrate each component with examples from this research.

Participatory action research approach

The goal of PAR is to create social change while generating theoretical and practical knowledge. It differs from more conventional research methodology in three ways: in its understanding and use of knowledge; its relationship with research participants; and, the introduction of change into the research process (Hockley *et al.*, 2005). Methodologically, the participants collaborate on all aspects of the research process and control research activities in the field setting (Cashman *et al.*, 2008). Knowledge is co-created by the researchers and participants through a reflective spiral of activity: identifying a problem;

planning a change; acting and observing the process and consequences of the change; reflecting on these processes and consequences; and re-planning, acting, observing, and reflecting (repeating the cycle) (Kemmis and McTaggart, 2000; 2005). Throughout the research, the change process and its outcomes are documented.

In our research, a PAR approach is appropriate because our goal is to change processes of care for dying residents and develop palliative care programmes. Using PAR recognizes the expertise of LTC home staff, residents, and families and promotes integration of the LTC communities' values and practices into palliative care. The LTC staff are co-researchers and they participate in creating and implementing all interventions. Meetings of the LTC palliative care teams are attended by the researchers and are used to generate knowledge. The knowledge created includes practical strategies for providing palliative care in LTC, as well as a greater theoretical understanding of the capacity development process that may be applicable to LTC homes nationally and internationally.

As long as the purpose and principles of PAR are respected, the research can use any form of data collection that researchers and participants determine are relevant for their study. In the project, our environmental assessment included: surveys, interviews, and focus groups, observations, document reviews of resident care records, and organizational analysis. We gathered data from residents, families, volunteers, and staff performing all roles within LTC, and community partners. We sought data about perceived quality of life and care, organizational culture, staff sense of empowerment, knowledge of palliative care, current care practices, communication, and relationships within the LTC home. Gathering multiple forms of data was appropriate since our goal was to 'get the story right'. Having multiple types of data and multiple sources of data enabled a more complete understanding and thus provided greater rigour in the research.

The depth and richness of the data also allowed us to appreciate the complexity of change that would be required to achieve our goal of implementing palliative care programmes. The data allowed the researchers and staff to identify multiple interventions encompassing the physical, social, psychological, spiritual, and practical aspects of palliative care as well as targeting changes for residents, families, direct care staff, and managers. Many interventions involved direct care staff, while others were implemented by managers or with community partners. Staff prioritized and gradually began to implement and evaluate the interventions using established organizational approaches to quality improvement, such as using plan-do-study-act cycles. Researchers also collected process and outcome data in conjunction with the LTC staff. As an example, the personal support workers (PSWs) generated the idea of providing 'comfort bags' for families of residents who were dying that consisted of toiletries, activities (such as crossword puzzles), and informational pamphlets on end-of-life issues. In a series of palliative care team meetings, the content, timing, and method of offering the comfort bags was modified until staff were satisfied with the result. Researchers participated in these discussions and documented the transformation of the intervention over time.

In PAR much is outside the control of the researchers because research progress is dependent on the participants, and the work occurs in a field setting that is subject to many internal and external forces that can interrupt plans (Kemmis and McTaggart, 2000; 2005; Prince and Kelley, 2010). Managing environmental impacts becomes an important part of the research process, and researchers must remain flexible. In our project, the LTC homes have coped with new regulatory legislation and requirements, a new electronic charting system, as well as changes in senior management which temporarily took their focus away from the palliative care project. Our project expectations needed to adapt to these realities and, whenever possible, synergies with other requirements were identified. For example, the new legislation mandated that LTC homes provide palliative care education and develop a pain management programme. The researchers identified how developing the palliative care programme could support the homes to meet these requirements.

In PAR, knowledge transfer to all stakeholders and participants is embedded in the process (Kemmis and McTaggart, 2000; 2005). Throughout our project, the first dissemination of research findings was always to the LTC staff participants which also helped to ensure that our interpretations were correct. This was done via organized presentations, workshops, and meetings. Subsequently, conference presentations have included our LTC partners as authors and presenters. Long-term care staff prepare articles for the project website, newsletters, and author manuals for the tool kit. This has the benefit of ensuring that the language and presentation of our research findings meets the needs of the primary audience, that is, staff of other LTC homes.

The focus of PAR is social change; such change may take a long time and maintaining participants' motivation is very important (Kemmis and McTaggart, 2000; 2005; Prince and Kelley, 2010). In our five-year project, researchers focused on creating quick benefits for the staff, such as meeting their requests for palliative care education. Research staff built personal relationships with the staff by spending time in the LTC homes; personal relationships enhanced engagement in the project. Researchers attended monthly meetings with the staff in the LTC homes and maintained ongoing email communications and telephone contact. As the project progressed over time, staff observed progress in creating the palliative care programme which served to sustain their motivation.

Researchers in PAR function as facilitators and catalysts in a change process that is controlled by the participants. This catalyst role is also consistent with the model of capacity development that requires changes to be generated from within the community and not imposed by external people or organizations. This next section describes four phases of the capacity development model created through previous research in rural communities (Kelley, 2007; Kelley *et al.*, 2011) and adapted for use in this research, since we view LTC homes as geographic and relational communities.

Capacity development model

Capacities are the collective capabilities found within and among people, organizations, and community networks and society (Norton *et al.*, 2002). From this perspective, we viewed LTC homes as communities that have the capacity to tackle their problems through collective problem-solving. Capacity development requires a long-term investment as it involves holistic change and is slow (Bolger, 2000). In our project, the researchers were committed to five years of involvement because they understood a major culture change would be needed for staff and LTC homes to fully embrace a new identity and role as providers of palliative care.

Capacity development promotes change from within each home and does not impose solutions from outside (Morgan, 1998). It focuses on: existing strengths and empowerment; the use of bottom-up, community-determined agendas and actions; and, processes for developing competence (Raeburn *et al.*, 2006). Our project offered resources to support this internal change process; for example, research assistants, graduate students, and money to purchase staff time for programme development. One PSW in each LTC home immediately joined the research team as a staff liaison, to guide and assist in the project. The capacity development model, depicted below in Figure 4.2, guided the PAR used to implement the four phases of developing palliative care for LTC.

Kelley's capacity development model is essentially a theory of change that depicts a 'bottom-up' community change process to develop palliative care programmes in four sequential phases:

Phase 1. Having sufficient antecedent conditions to begin the change process.

Phase 2. Experiencing a catalyst for change.

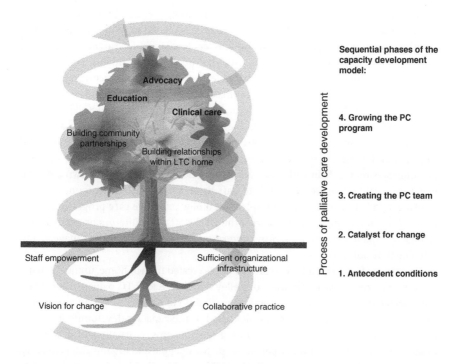

Fig. 4.2 Capacity development model for long-term care.
Adapted with permission from Mary Lou Kelley, Developing Rural Communities' Capacity for Palliative Care: a Conceptual Model. *Journal of Palliative Care* (Autumn 2007), **23**(3): 147, copyright © Institut universitaire de gériatrie de Montréal, 2007.

Phase 3. Creating a palliative care team.

Phase 4. Growing the palliative care programme.

This model was applied to build capacity in the LTC home. Using PAR, the phases were initiated sequentially by the LTC home staff, but the overall development process was dynamic and non-linear, shaped by internal and external forces. At each phase of the model, there were strategies to guide the LTC staff to manage challenges such as lack of resources, internal resistance to palliative care, and bureaucracy. Research interventions in the LTC home respected enabling factors identified in the model: being focused on the whole organization; educating providers; working together; internal leadership; and participants taking pride in their accomplishments. Ultimately, by implementing the model, the LTC home staff created a comprehensive palliative care programme that provided clinical care, education, and advocacy; built relationships within the LTC home; and made strong community partnerships with outside expert resources (QPC-LTC Alliance, 2010). We next describe the implementation process that occurred in the PAR research.

Prior to initiating the PAR research, researchers assessed each LTC home's antecedent conditions for change through a comprehensive environmental assessment (Phase 1 of Kelley's model). Antecedent conditions for change are: collaborative practice; sufficient organizational infrastructure; having a vision for change; and staff sense of empowerment. Understanding these conditions for LTC homes required the researchers to understand current values, attitudes, and practices related to palliative care and to identify strengths, gaps, facilitators, and barriers to change. Researchers conducted surveys, interviews, and focus groups with staff in all roles, residents, families, and community partners. Observations and reviews of resident care records and policy were also completed. These data were summarized by the research team.

Initiating the PAR involved creating a catalyst for change (Phase 2 of Kelley's model) in each LTC home. Researchers shared the findings of the environmental assessment with Alliance members, long-term care home managers, staff, and families to build common understanding of current capacity and identify goals for change. A strategic planning session was held with LTC staff in each home to discuss their own data and plan the palliative care programme. The staff vision for change laid the foundation for creating a palliative care team to implement a new palliative care programme. The research team continued to work with the LTC staff as facilitators or catalysts for change by organizing meetings, providing resources, advocating with managers, and teaching new skills.

An inter-professional palliative care team was created in each home, uniquely structured to the homes' wishes (Phase 3 of Kelley's model). Each LTC palliative care team then created their palliative care programme (Phase 4 of Kelley's model) incorporating interventions in the five categories identified in the capacity development model: clinical care, education, advocacy, building relationships internally within the LTC home, and building community partnerships with people and organizations to assist them in providing palliative care. Each LTC home identified their unique priority interventions to be implemented and evaluated together by researchers and staff. At the time of writing, 23 interventions are completed or underway, such as new pain assessment protocols, new palliative care policy, staff and family education programmes, and new partnerships with hospice volunteer visitors. The interventions are being shared throughout the Alliance via bi-annual meetings and at the end of the project the most successful interventions will be included in a tool kit for LTC homes developing palliative care programmes. The model thus outlines an incremental process for PAR where the right resources are provided at the right time when they are most applicable.

Our developing understanding of how a researcher 'does' PAR and 'capacity development' is addressed in the next section of the chapter, with examples from the research.

The four practice principles of participatory action research

In our project, we achieved change while respecting the philosophy of PAR (Kemmis and McTaggart, 2000; 2005) and capacity development (Kelley, 2007) through adopting four practice principles in our work: cultural competence, empowerment, relational ethics, and partnerships. These practice principles have evolved from the core values of social work, the professional discipline of the authors (CASW, 2010).

Empowerment

In our research we defined empowerment as the state of feeling you have with the control over your own destiny. In the workplace it includes the ability to think, behave, take action, and control your work and decision making in autonomous ways (Palliative Alliance, 2010). Our environmental assessment data indicated that while PSWs have the most intimate knowledge of the needs of their dying residents and their families and do the majority of the day-to-day care, they do not perceive themselves to have much influence in care planning and decision-making (QPC-LTC Alliance, 2010). It was thus clear from the beginning of this research that empowerment of the PSWs was key to the development of palliative care in LTC. We also knew that the success of the PAR process depended on PSW investment in the process of organizational change. The researchers' focus was on the PSW experience, making an explicit statement that we valued their experience and knowledge. Engaging the PSWs in the research as experts and advisors was contrary to the usual knowledge hierarchy where the more educated nurses and physicians are more respected.

In a focus group we conducted in the third year of this research, the PSWs talked about how their involvement in the research led them to trust their own instincts and knowledge: 'We've learned things just by experience alone. There's nothing wrong with being confident and saying those things.' They talked about having discovered a sense of voice: 'Being able to voice those things because we always felt like we weren't allowed to before', as well as a strong sense of professional identity: 'We're not registered, but we're still professionals.' They told us they were speaking up more regularly and more confidently with registered nursing staff, and were seeing communication barriers and professional silos beginning to break down.

Personal support workers now saw themselves as 'in the driver's seat' and recognized that: 'As a PSW I am sitting in the front seat of that change right now. I feel empowered by it.' One of the PSWs said that 'Before this [research] started happening I felt like I was at the bottom of the healthcare totem pole. Now I am a little bit okay with saying that I may be near the bottom but I am a stable base . . . right?' Another PSW said: 'We're not the bottom. We're the front line.' This reframing of their position as 'the stable base' or as 'the front line' expressed their growing sense of identity, pride, and power.

The PSWs also discovered their power as a group: 'If we stick together . . . what are they going to do, fight all of us? It's something that we believe in so strongly that we are sticking together!' They talked about forming a PSW network with the idea of having regular meetings to problem solve together. Finally, they talked about how being empowered had made them better PSWs, happier and more purposeful; and they talked about how this had transformed their workplace: 'You're coming into work more empowered, happier . . . you bring that to this building, to these people.'

However, empowerment also came with some risks for the PSWs. With their newly-discovered sense of voice came a rebalancing of power in the institutional hierarchy which they experienced as both exciting and risky. They expressed worry that they might inadvertently overstep the mark and that their new found solidarity might meet with retribution. Their vulnerability in the organization thus surfaced as an ethical issue for the researchers and participants to problem solve together.

Relational ethics

Relational ethics is the second practice principle and is vital to managing the unfolding dynamics of this capacity development process. A relational ethics stance calls attention to the interpersonal nature of the PAR research contract, and the ongoing need for maintenance of that interpersonal contract through continuous dialogue and joint problem solving about all aspects of the research. Relational ethics requires human engagement, mutual respect, embodiment of lived experience, and creation of an ethical environment for action (Bergum and Dossetor, 2005). It is an ethic of action that focuses on *how* we treat one another and ourselves rather than *why* we act. For research, the usual way of thinking about ethics approvals (where participants and researchers agree in advance on all the details, and then 'sign off' on de-contextualized consent documents) is not appropriate. Instead, we need to think about consent as a dynamic process of ongoing collaboration and working out of details as they unfold in real time and in real place.

A relational ethical stance means researchers and participants are both experts. The researchers bring their knowledge, contacts, and networks. The participants, their deep knowing of the community they represent, and their aspirations for the research. Together they forge a partnership where areas of moral concern are negotiated as they arise, through mutual learning and accommodation (Bergum and Dossetor, 2005).

Cultural competency

Culture implies the integrated pattern of behaviour that includes thoughts, communications, actions, customs, beliefs, values, and institutions of a social group (NASW, 2001; Prince and Kelley, 2010). We include cultural competency as the third practice principle of PAR because researchers will commonly be working within a social group whose experience and perspectives are different to their own. In our project, we understand

LTC as a unique culture with rules, constraints, customs, and patterns of interaction and communication that are understood best by the people who work there.

For researchers to successfully engage in a new culture requires the same sensitivities one would need to engage in professional practice with any unfamiliar culture: self-awareness and a commitment to understanding our own personal, cultural, and professional values; respect for and appreciation of multicultural identities; and gaining appropriate knowledge and skills to understand and behave respectfully in the culture (NASW, 2001). Our experience as professional social workers and PAR researchers tells us that successful engagement is facilitated by an attitude of curiosity about cultural differences, genuine willingness to learn, and openness to authentic dialogue.

Being culturally competent in LTC means appreciating the ecology of constraints within which the staff work. There are so many things over which they have no control: governing legislation and funding, union contracts, professional scopes of practice, and health system dynamics such as the shortage of acute care beds or changes to home care provision. Cultural competence means acknowledging that LTC staff members are themselves the experts on their culture, and taking time to learn from them. It also means that we have to earn their trust, and we do this by safeguarding our commitment to joint decision making and safety for all participants. The culture change they are trying to make can only be successful if it is grafted onto their culture and ecology of constraints.

Partnerships

When thinking of capacity building as a set of skills, resources, and knowledge held within a whole network or community of partners, not just within one individual or LTC home, then a key strategy in capacity building is the development of new partnerships. Partnerships are perhaps one of the most important things researchers have to offer in PAR, that is, a network of people and resources that can help participants achieve their vision of becoming palliative care centres of excellence.

In our research, the Quality Palliative Care in Long Term Care Alliance (QPC-LTC Alliance, 2010) was created as a partnership of LTC homes, researchers, and community organizations. Alliance partners (for example the Alzheimer's Society, or hospice volunteers) bring an infusion of palliative care knowledge and expertise from the wider community into LTC. They help break down the institutional silos that have marginalized LTC homes and made them resource-poor. They place LTC homes back in the wider community. These partnerships will last long after the research is over, and should help sustain LTC culture change into the future. Indeed, one of the strategies for making culture change sustainable after completion of the research is to make partnership-building a core strategy in PAR. This is the rationale for developing the researcher, LTC home, and community partner alliance at the outset of the project.

There are several challenges in forging such partnerships. One is to overcome the institutionalized norm of 'we can do it all ourselves' and the fear and uncertainty surrounding bringing people in from the outside. Another is that potential partners from outside organizations come with different cultural norms and practices and may not know how to adapt what they do to the culture of LTC. They may be locked into existing resources and unable to imagine expanding their role or mandate. Or quite simply, neither side may know how to make the first step. Here we see the interrelatedness of the principles in our integrative framework: cultural competence, that is, a deep under-standing of the culture of LTC, and, an ethic of mutual trust between researchers and LTC participants, are absolutely crucial for these partnerships to get started and to flourish. The researchers are like cultural brokers, facilitating the transfer and integra-tion of practices and expertise from new partners, and the building of an extended community. In our PAR project 43 different community partners have committed to supporting LTC homes in their transition to developing palliative care. Some are clini-cal partners, others provide palliative care education, and others serve a knowledge translation function. However, the common purpose is to build capacity for better pal-liative care by building community partnerships.

Our experience has been that acceptance of outside partners has increased as the PSWs have become more empowered. The more capable and assured they become in their own role, and the more empowered they are to articulate that role, the better able they are to enter any exchange as full and equal partners. An interesting example arose when there was an opportunity to partner with the local hospice volunteer organiza-tion. The PSWs were protective of the residents and did not know if they could trust the volunteers who were, after all, strangers. Furthermore, the PSWs longed to be the ones at the bedside when their residents were dying; it was not a simple matter for them to turn over these precious moments to outside volunteers. As the PSWs increas-ingly found their voice they were able to articulate their concerns about this proposed partnership. They could easily have let the partnership fail, but instead they were able to negotiate a mutually agreeable resolution. It was decided that the volunteers would be assigned to the PSW rather than to the resident; that way the PSWs would have more say in what the volunteers did at the bedside. It was an outcome that reinforced for the researchers how important the empowerment of the PSWs truly was to the suc-cess of the whole research project.

Conclusion

The purpose of this chapter has been to propose an integrative framework that is being used in PAR to create palliative care programmes in LTC homes. The components of the framework integrate synergistically and their values and principles complement one another. Both capacity development and PAR represent a commitment to com-munity and participant control, and creating social change that benefits them. The practice principles of empowerment, cultural competency, relational ethics, and part-nerships operationalize how we as researchers can 'do PAR' in a way that is genuine and respectful of our participants. In our experience, all the elements of this frame-work are equally important and reinforce one another.

While this chapter has focused on using PAR to develop palliative care in LTC homes, the authors believe that our framework could apply to any research focusing on palliative care capacity development in a defined community or organization. The four-phase capacity development model is a theory of change that is independent of any particular socio-cultural context, and builds on the local people and resources. Combined with PAR as a methodological approach, this framework thus has potential as an international resource.

References

Bergum, V. and Dossetor, J. (2005) *Relational Ethics: The Full Meaning of Respect*. Maryland: University Publishing Group Inc.

Bolger, J. (2000) *Capacity Development: Why, What and How*. Gatineau (QC): CIDA, Policy Branch; (Capacity development occasional series 1, no. 1).

CASW (2010) *Canadian Association of Social Workers: Guidelines for Ethical Practice*. Available at http://www.casw-acts.ca/en/what-social-work/casw-code-ethics (accessed 18 March 2012).

Casarett, D.J., Hirschman, K.B., and Henry, M.R. (2001) Does Hospice Have a Role in Nursing Home Care at the End of Life? *Journal of the American Geriatrics Society*, 49: 1493–8.

Cashman, S., Adeky, B.S., Allen, A.J., et al. (2008) The Power and the Promise: Working with Communities to Analyze Data, Interpret Findings, And Get To Outcomes. *American Journal of Public Health*, 98: 1407–17.

Ferris, F.D., Balfour, H.M., Bowen, K., *et al.* (2002) *A Model to Guide Hospice Palliative Care*. Ottawa, ON: Canadian Hospice Palliative Care Association. Available at: http://www.market-marche.chpca.net/chpca/marketplace.nsf/prodnum/0605ecd/$file/a+model+to+guide+hospice+palliative+care+2002-urlupdate-august2005.pdf (accessed 27 January 2012).

Foner, N. (1995) *The Caregiving Dilemma: Work in an American Nursing Home*. Berkeley: University of California Press.

Hockley, J., Dewar, B., and Watson, J. (2005) Promoting End-of-Life Care in Nursing Homes Using an 'Integrated Care Pathway for the Last Days of Life'. *Journal of Research in Nursing*, **10**: 135–52.

Kelley, M.L. (2007) Developing Rural Communities' Capacities for Palliative Care: A Conceptual Model. *Journal of Palliative Care*, **23**: 143–53.

Kelley, M.L., Williams, A., DeMiglio, L., and Mettam, H. (2011) Developing Rural Palliative Care: Validating a Conceptual Model. *Rural and Remote Health*, 11: 1717.

Kemmis, S. and McTaggart, R. (2000) Participatory Action Research. In: N.K. Denzin, and Y.S. Lincoln (eds), *The Sage Handbook of Qualitative Research*, 2nd edn, pp. 567–606. Thousand Oaks: Sage.

Kemmis, S. and McTaggart, R. (2005) Participatory Action Research. In: N.K. Denzin, Y.S. Lincoln (eds), *The Sage Handbook of Qualitative Research*, 3rd edn, pp. 559–604. Thousand Oaks: Sage.

Ley, D.C. (1989) The elderly and palliative care. *Journal of Palliative Care*, **5**: 43–5.

Ministry of Health and Long-Term Care (2007) *Long-Term Care Homes Act, 2007*. Available at: http://www.health.gov.on.ca/english/public/legislation/ltc_homes/ltc_homes.html (accessed 27 January 2012).

Morgan, P. (1998) *Capacity and Capacity Development: Some Strategies*. Hull (QC): CIDA, Policy Branch.

National Association of Social Workers (NASW) (2001) *National Association of Social Workers: Standards for Cultural Competence in Social Work Practice*. Available at: http://www.socialworkers.org/practice/standards/NASWCulturalStandards.pdf (accessed 27 January 2012).

Norton, B.L., McLeroy, K.R., Burdine, J.N., Felix, M.R.J., and Dorsey A.M. (2002) Community Capacity: Concept, Theory, and Methods. In: R.D. Clementi, R. Crosby, and M. Kegler (eds), *Emerging Theories in Health Promotion Practice and Research*. pp. 194–227. San Francisco: Jossey-Bass.

Palliative Alliance (2010) *Quality Palliative Care—Long-term Care Alliance.* Available at: www.palliativecarealliance.ca.

Prince, H. and Kelley, M.L. (2010) An Integrative Framework for Conducting Palliative Care Research with First Nations Communities. *Journal of Palliative Care*, 26: 47–53.

Quality Palliative Care in Long Term Care (QPC-LTC) Alliance (2010) *Quality Palliative Care in Long Term Care: Project results.* Available at: http://www.palliativealliance.ca/project-results (accessed 27 January 2012).

Raeburn, J., Akerman, M., Chuengsatiansup, K., Mejia, F., and Oladepo, O. (2006) Community Capacity Building and Health Promotion an a Globalized World. *Health Promotion*, 21: S84–90.

Reynolds, K., Henderson, M., Schulman, A., and Hanson, L.C. (2002) Needs of the Dying in Nursing Homes. *Journal of Palliative Medicine*, 5: 895–901.

Sachs, G.A., Shega, J.W., and Cox-Hayley, D. (2004) Barriers to Excellent End of Life Care for Patients with Dementia. *Journal of General Internal Medicine*, 19(10): 1057–63.

Sims-Gould, J., Wiersma, E., Arseneau, L., et al. (2010) Care Provider Perspectives on End-of-life Care in Long-term Care Homes: Implications for Whole-Person and Palliative Care. *Journal of Palliative Care*, 26: 122–9.

Wowchuk, S.M., McClement, S., and Bond, J. (2006) The Challenge of Providing Palliative Care in the Nursing Home: Part 1: External Factors. *International Journal of Palliative Nursing*, 12: 260–7.

Wowchuk, S.M., McClement, S., and Bond, J. (2007) The Challenge of Providing Palliative Care in the Nursing Home Part 2: Internal Factors. *International Journal of Palliative Nursing*, 13: 345–50.

Chapter 5

First, second, and third person inquiry

Geralyn Hynes

Introduction

Action research is underpinned by practice-based knowledge development and with a focus on addressing problems in their everyday context. Thus, action research extends beyond and should be differentiated from change management. In action research there is an emphasis on contribution to knowledge development, both through and alongside a change in practice that arises from a practice-based problem focus. For Coghlan and Brannick the: 'Desired outcomes of the action research approach are not just solutions to the immediate problems but important learning from outcomes, both intended and unintended, and a contribution to scientific knowledge and theory. In the case of change management, there is little or no emphasis on knowledge development and contribution to the field' (Coghlan and Brannick, 2010: 5).

Action research is grounded in lived experience, and collaboration and partnership (Bradbury and Reason, 2003). In other words, action research is concerned with our everyday experiences and people's rights to have a say in what and how knowledge is generated about them (Reason, 2006). The privileging of practice-based knowledge and lived experiences, how we attend to democratic principles in our inquiry, and how we mediate different views and experiences among different stakeholders, are all value-laden and political (see Chapter 15). These groundings are captured in different theoretical perspectives from within the broad church of action research. By way of example, Shani and Passmore (1985), see the theory of action research as framed within four factors, namely: contextual factors; quality of relationships; quality of the action research process; and the outcomes of the action research effort.

A further key distinguishing feature of action research is that it is conducted in the present and is future oriented (Chandler and Torbert, 2003). Other forms of research are retrospective, whether this is seeking people's accounts of experiences (that have already occurred) or measuring an outcome. How we interrogate the values we bring to bear on the inquiry process alongside an iterative questioning approach to our practice in the moment are addressed through the idea of first, second, and third person inquiry.

In this chapter, I will outline how first, second, and third person inquiry is defined and understood from different theoretical perspectives within the action research literature. In the final section I will outline the challenges of first, second, and third person inquiry with particular reference to palliative care research and practice development.

Definition for first, second, and third person inquiry

First person action research addresses the researcher's inward inquiry, mindfulness, and reflection. Second person inquiry addresses inquiry with others, while third person inquiry looks to extend outwards from single case/project inquiries towards creating greater impact, for example through building or connecting with networks of inquiry.

First person inquiry

First person inquiry addresses the researcher's skills in attending to the moment and the choices that are made in responding to information or engagement on a moment-by-moment basis. Since action research takes a purposive approach towards addressing the value laden nature of inquiry, how the researcher hears and responds to points always affects choices being made in the moment. First person inquiry brings to the fore the individual researcher's own engagement with the world and its impact on others. Coghlan and Brannick (2010) refer to an intended self study of the researcher in action. Judi Marshall (2004: 309) describes first person inquiry as: 'Both an approach to inquiry in itself—as I research my own practice—and, in my view, foundational to overtly collaborative forms of research'. In this way, in first person inquiry we become mindful of our engagement with issues such as power, different worldviews, and unquestioned truths that underpin our practice.

For Reason and Torbert (2001), first person inquiry fosters mindfulness, taking us 'upstream' where inquiry is directed towards basic assumptions and 'the source of our attention (showing, for example, how our particular habits of thought sometimes facilitate and other times cut us off from ongoing experiential knowing)' (Reason and Torbert, 2001: 12). Travelling upstream brings clarity to the 'whys and what' we are trying to achieve in our research both for ourselves as individuals, and others. First person inquiry also brings us 'downstream' to examine our everyday behaviour and the impact of our actions. Downstream addresses 'the congruence or incongruence of one's behaviour with purposes or espoused theories' (Reason and Torbert, 2001: 13).

What Marshall (2004), and Reason and Torbert (2001) have in common is a view of first person inquiry not as a discrete element of action research, but rather, as a stance or attitude of inquiry towards engagement with the every day. In other words, first person inquiry is a way of being in the inquiry process. Coghlan (2008: 352) refers to his: 'Approach in the philosophical practice of first person inquiry, thereby positioning my understanding of authenticity (a term usually used to connote qualities like being genuine and true to values) in an appropriation of how I experience, understand, judge, and act in my life, and particularly in action research' (Coghlan, 2008: 352). This sets first person inquiry as fundamental to an inquiry process that seeks to question or free oneself from the restricted forces of the 'taken for granted' assumptions of one's world.

First person inquiry then, is both 'reflection in action' and 'reflection on action' that recognizes that we are continually taking stances or positions in how we hear others, understand our world, and articulate our purposes. Where action research is both value-laden and seeks to confront the values that underpin our everyday practice, first person inquiry is the means by which the action researcher begins by confronting his/her basic and often untested assumptions. However, though viewed by many action researchers as fundamental to their research, first person inquiry is about one's relationship with the world and others. Thus, first person inquiry begins not with self alone, but rather self *with* other.

This reflects living life as inquiry or what Wicks *et al.* refer to as the thoughtful integration of 'various theoretical perspectives and life experiences' (Wicks *et al.*, 2008: 15) that shape our being in the world as action researchers. Not unrelated is the idea of action research as living theory (Whitehead and McNiff, 2006), which invites practitioners to define and make known for others the judgements against which they judge their own work. These different perspectives have in common the view that action research begins with first person inquiry.

Second person inquiry

Second person inquiry is inquiry with others through face-to-face dialogue on issues of shared interest or concern, focusing on the development of interpersonal dialogue and applying planning, action, and reflection cycles to the process. In action research literature, second person inquiry attracts the most attention and appears to have the most immediate impact in terms of changes in practice. Typically, a group of people come together to address a shared interest in an issue or problem through applying iterative cycles of constructing, planning, action, and evaluation (Coghlan and Brannick, 2010).

These cycles are intended to challenge taken for granted assumptions, the gap between espoused theories, and theories in action (Argyris, 2006) establishing participative and democratic principles that are fundamental to action research. However, second person inquiry is fraught with difficulties, particularly in healthcare action research. A group of people with a shared interest, for example nurses working in palliative care, will share a set of values and language that is specific to their world of palliative care and professional position within healthcare. For such a homogenous group, questioning assumptions and values about practice can be difficult and give rise to errors of consensus collusion (Reason, 2006) in which the group defends its version of reality and does not engage in alternatives. Errors of consensus collusion may also lead to a strong sense of identity which can in turn lead to an 'us and them' view of the world.

Second person inquiry in healthcare action research is more commonly an open-boundary inquiry (Heron, 1996). Open-boundary inquiries are those in which the inquiry group extends the inquiry beyond the group itself. Put simply, if an inquiry group comprised of healthcare professionals decides to survey or collect experiences of patients this is an open-boundary inquiry. If such an inquiry group does not include patients, the group is then engaging in research *on* rather than *with* people. Moreover, if the inquiry group is espousing the principle that people who are the target of an inquiry have a right to say what and how knowledge is generated about them, then that principle is breached by an open-boundary inquiry.

The challenges of group homogeneity and open-boundary inquiries are addressed through a strong focus on confronting the important power differential within a group, and between the group and others who are targeted by or part of the inquiry process.

In particular, the quality of the inquiry is addressed through recognizing and making explicit choices that are made throughout the process in relation to practical focus, knowledge generation, and participation. Recent discussions in the action research literature have highlighted paradoxes that can surface when seeking to create conditions or space for opening conversations towards mutual understanding (Arieli *et al.*, 2009; Ospina *et al.*, 2004; Wicks and Reason, 2009). In reporting on their experiences Arieli *et al.* (2009) illustrate that however experienced and enthusiastic facilitators and group participants might be, establishing an environment or space for mutual understanding is particularly challenging.

For the facilitator or lead action researcher, a particular challenge is how to create an environment for articulating and developing the skills for inquiry while also seeking to transfer ownership of the inquiry to the group. Wicks and Reason (2009) refer to this as opening a 'communicative space' in which the group must struggle with desire for action while still uncertain about how to begin. An important mediating force is an individuals' capacity to engage in examining their individual positionality and worldview, and relationship with the group through first person inquiry. Arieli *et al.* (2009) offer a number of approaches aimed at addressing and making discussable embedded gaps in power and cultural differences. These include: sharing resources; attending to demands for action early on; prompt engagement with conflicts about roles, tasks, boundaries, and authority; attending to joint reflection and value-based nature of individual reasoning; and, taking the initiative to admit errors.

Third person inquiry

Third person inquiry looks to extend outwards from single case/project inquiries towards creating greater impact, for example through building or connecting with networks of inquiry. At its simplest, third person inquiry is about dissemination: action researchers bringing their projects to a wider audience or writing about action research such as I am doing here. At a deeper level, however, third person inquiry may be much more than dissemination. Gustavsen amongst others (Gustavsen, 2003a; 2003b; Reason, 2003) has debated the importance of moving beyond 'the single case'. In other words, the scope of action research will be limited if it is viewed only in terms of individual projects. There needs to be a conversation between projects so that they are connected. Connected in this sense is not about sharing the same topic but rather that there is a wider conversation or social movement about action research.

Third person inquiry presents significant challenges to action researchers. Relating project narratives, the choices made in respect to participation, opening a space for inquiry, first person inquiry, etc., is not easily done within the constraints of research and clinical journals or indeed, a 15-minute oral presentation at a research conference. We are challenged to find ways of engaging with a wider audience that allow an opening for conversations about practice in the context of action research.

Many projects involve all three forms of inquiry (Chandler and Torbert, 2003; Marshall, 2004; Reason and Bradbury, 2006; 2008a) reflecting the argument that, 'the most compelling and enduring kind of action research will engage all three strategies' (Reason and Bradbury, 2008a: 6).

Different perspectives on first, second, and third person inquiry

Chandler and Torbert (2003) describe how first, second, and third person inquiry can occur in the past, present, and future. By this they mean that an action research's departure point begins in the past (what has happened) but takes place in the present, and seeks to shape the future. Researching in the present draws attention to: how we become present in the moment or attentive to what is happening; how we perceive what is happening; how we are forming judgements about what is happening; how we are acting; and, our intentions which are future oriented. This 'present in the moment' is done at the levels of first, second, and third person inquiry.

Marshall and Reason (2007) name an attitude of inquiry in which the inquirer is present in the moment, questioning and testing her assumptions and sense-making, but at the same time being open to contradictions and engaging with the emergent nature of the research process. It is this attitude of inquiry that brings a first person inquiry dimension to all aspects of an inquiry. Marshall (2006) describes her first person inquiry as consisting of three elements:

1. Holding together inner and outer arcs of attention as in attending to one's own perceiving and assumptions (inner arc), and questioning or testing, possibly with others, one's assumptions, sense-making, or ideas.
2. Attending to cycles of action and reflection.
3. Being both active and receptive, for example in testing one's own sense-making.

Through an inner arc of attention, Marshall (2006) describes how she observes herself drawing meaning, framing issues, and choosing when and how to speak at a given moment. This also draws attention to the assumptions she makes and the patterns of her utterances. This requires note-taking and attending to that which is 'selected' for noting. Outer arcs of attention involve raising and questioning issues, and testing assumptions with others. This draws attention to how one presents or frames points, and reacts to other perspectives expressed within an inquiry group. Through her inner and outer arcs of attention, Marshall opens up her own sense-making, values, and attitudes to scrutiny. In so doing, it is possible to recognize subtle choices that are being made in the moment over the course of the inquiry process. Put simply, attending to how we choose, frame, and respond to points being raised helps to question the values we ascribe to them.

In a more recent work, Coghlan (2008) draws on the notion of authenticity and the work of Bernard Lonergan, a Canadian theologian and philosopher, through which he (Coghlan) engages in action research. Authenticity in this sense refers to recognizing or grasping how one experiences situations, understands, judges, and acts. This provides the structure for enacting action research. Here, Coghlan introduces authenticity in the context of quality in the researcher. This is a departure from the more typical view of authenticity in research in relation to its association with quality in terms of data. For Coghlan (2008), different ways of knowing or understanding the world, such as those highlighted by action research scholars (Reason and Bradbury, 2008b) all involve experiencing, understanding, and judging. He positions inquiry in action research in relation to the structure of knowing. We understand 'how' and 'what' we know through experience, understanding, and judgement.

Attending to experience, understanding, and judgement which lead to action, offers us the means to better understand and scrutinize our sense-making. We do this through attentiveness, intelligence, and reasonableness in self-reflection, which Coghlan compares with the requirements for inference testing proposed by Argyris (1995) in action science, and framing our speech in development inquiry proposed by Torbert (1999). Different approaches within action research such as action science and development action inquiry offer various techniques for testing assumptions, attentiveness, and inferences. Authenticity involves (Coghlan, 2008):

◆ Being open to the experience of the data before us—so we must be attentive.

◆ Questioning and wondering about what is before us—so we must bring our intelligence to bear.

◆ Examining and testing what we hold to be the case—so we must be reasonable.

◆ Discerning what is the best way forward, being sensitive to the choices we make—so we must be responsible.

The point here is that authenticity provides a frame for self-reflective practice in both first and second person action research. As with Marshall's arcs of attention and the work of others referred to above, authenticity draws attention to the inter-dependence of first, second, and third person in action research. The role of self in action research cannot be separated from how an action research group constructs and addresses the problems that are targeted in an inquiry and subsequently reported through third person inquiry. Thus first, second, and third person inquiry are also first, second, and third person practice. It is this idea of practice or enacting action research that Coghlan (2008) addresses as authenticity.

Single and double loop learning

First and second person inquiry bring attention to values underpinning our practice. Questions arising from actions shift from 'what worked' to examining the value of the things we are seeking to achieve; those that are obvious and those which are less so. The rationale for an action research initiative may typically be to address a problem. Single loop learning occurs when a problem is addressed while holding to existing values, attitudes, and frameworks. Double loop learning occurs when underlying values, attitudes, norms, and frameworks are tackled and modified (Argyris, 2006). For Argyris (2006) double loop learning is necessary for organizational learning to take place. In other words, with double loop learning, basic ideas, policies, and strategies are confronted and their values are scrutinized. For Coghlan and Casey, how individual action research projects impact on, 'what and how a hospital learns depends on strategies of aggregating individual learning to team and interdepartmental group, and organizational learning' (Coghlan and Casey, 2001: 680).

Different action research approaches carry with them a strong emphasis on making sense of existing practice through a critical lens that questions attention to different voices, mindfulness in the moment, and interrogating embedded culture. It is these characteristics that bring double loop learning to the fore in developing practice. Action research thus provides a framework for developing practice in a manner that recognizes the role and responsibility of the individual through first person inquiry, while also inviting those involved to engage fully and critically in the process through second person inquiry.

Developing practice to address palliative care needs of a given patient group requires: awareness raising; development and implementation of processes for referral and consultancy practices and care pathways; communication within and between different care teams, disciplines, and services; and knowledge and skills development to address specific clinical practice and care issues for different patient cohorts. In other words, developing practice to address palliative care needs requires changes in practice and development of palliative care knowledge. For this to be realized, double loop learning is an essential ingredient.

Challenges of first, second, and third person inquiry with reference to palliative care research and practice development

Having outlined some of the key theoretical principles and perspectives in relation to first, second, and third person inquiry, let us turn to particular challenges that confront action researchers who seek to develop palliative care practice. This final section addresses four broad challenges, namely those related to:

1. Engagement and participation.
2. Balancing an open-boundary inquiry in healthcare.
3. Addressing the potential conflict between acute/continuing philosophies of care on the one hand and, on the other, a palliative care approach through double loop learning.
4. Improving capacity of individual projects to have wider influence through third person inquiry.

Engagement and participation

Enshrined in the WHO definition for palliative care (Sepúlveda *et al.*, 2002) is the emphasis on supporting the patient and family throughout a final illness. While this understanding is not without its critics (Randall and Downie, 2006), it remains the most frequently cited definition in research and policy documents. Implicit in this definition is the strong partnership between the palliative care healthcare professional and the patient and family. Even Randall and Downie (2006), strong critics of the WHO palliative care definition, make explicit the need to address patients' views about their values and goals. Different definitions seem in agreement that palliative care connects with an understanding of the illness experience, namely: how patients engage with and make judgements about how best to cope with or endure the distress and problems in daily living. In other words, different kinds of knowledge are not only acknowledged but are integral to the patient's and family's palliative care. It follows, then, that related service development and evaluative research must find ways of engaging with patients' and families' experiences. Not surprisingly, there is increasing interest in the contribution of action research to palliative care since the action researcher is focused on engaging with and acting upon different ways of understanding the world.

Nevertheless, action research faces serious challenges in palliative care. The open-ended and active participative nature of action research presents difficulties for ethics committees to support patient involvement for obvious reasons. For healthcare professionals, there are also practical constraints, including shift work and balancing meetings with managing the wide catchment area for those who provide community support. While palliative care services have long placed an emphasis on multi-disciplinary team working, developing multi-disciplinary action research groups may present with additional practical constraints.

Balancing an open-boundary inquiry in healthcare

John Heron (1996) drew attention to the significance of the boundaries within which an inquiry operates. Closed-boundary inquiries are those in which the action research group focus on inquiry from within the group. In other words, the inquiry process does not engage with people outside the group. Typically, a closed-boundary inquiry might involve the group members exploring practice. In contrast, open-boundary inquiries involve engagement with people not directly involved in the group (Heron and Reason, 2001). Open-boundary inquiries are challenged by a potential conflict between on the one hand, giving people the right to have a say in what and how knowledge is generated about them, while on the other hand generating data about them (Heron and Reason, 2001). Since action researchers place particular emphasis on participation, it follows that inquiry boundaries reflect the realization of participative goals. Reviews of action research in healthcare and nursing specifically raise concerns about the apparent limited patient participation (Munn-Giddings et al., 2008; Waterman et al., 2001). Against the practical constraints of gaining fuller participation, involving patients and different disciplines can be a difficult balancing act.

First person inquiry and practice as integral to second person inquiry provides an important mechanism for questioning current practices and the values underpinning them. Marshall's (2004) arcs of attention and Coghlan's (2008) authenticity, target engagement of self in moment-to-moment questioning and openness to other understandings of the world. Both offer the palliative care action researcher a framework for reconciling the limitations of uni-disciplinary inquiries and restricted patient engagement. Different approaches to action research offer theories to support first and second person inquires. Argyris's (2006) distinctions between espoused theories and theories in use, for example, draw attention to behaviour practices at individual and organizational levels.

Double loop learning in palliative care

Action research is becoming increasingly important in efforts to improve palliative care for patients with chronic illnesses in acute and residential care settings, as this book highlights. Despite policies in place supporting palliative care across care settings and disease groups, there are also concerns about failures in integrating palliative care into a generalist workload (Gott et al., 2012). Such failures are perhaps less surprising if understood in terms of single and double loop learning. Recent projects (Hockley and Froggatt, 2006) highlight the importance of attending to the values that underpin care at both individual and organizational levels. This reflects double loop learning. Conversely, for Gott *et al.* (2012), nurses were struggling to integrate palliative care in practice when organizational values had not been addressed. Put simply, integrating palliative care in generalist practice is not simply a process of adding another task to a working day. Rather, a philosophy of palliative care may fundamentally conflict with care practices in acute and residential care settings unless opportunity is given to clarify staff attitudes, values, and organizational frameworks.

Wider influence through third person inquiry

Much of the action research literature pays considerable attention to first and second person inquiry. Less attention in healthcare action research is given to third person inquiry theory. Third person action research reflects the process of taking an inquiry to a wider audience such as you, the reader, or through presentations at conferences. However, Gustavsen's (2003a) issue with the single case is pertinent to palliative care. Gustavsen argues the importance of networking in order for single cases to form a wider community of action research. This brings the significance of the single case beyond its narrow topic towards contributing to a social movement that seeks to promote action research principles. In other words the single palliative care project should be capable of influencing major challenges such as national policy implementation by generating and supporting conversations about action research.

One can also argue that third person inquiry is about continuing the conversation that emerged from the immediate project. Such a conversation if initiated in the spirit of action research might actively seek to engage with the principles of participation and knowledge co-production.

Conclusion

First, second, and third person inquiry underpins many of the current theoretical debates on action research. By attending to first person inquiry we bring to action research a focus on our individual values and beliefs, attentiveness to the voice of others, and engagement with the inquiry process. Second person inquiry represents most of the action research reported in healthcare. However, the strength of a second person inquiry in terms of double loop learning is contingent on the degree to which this can address values and beliefs, norms, and frameworks within practice.

Action research offers a potentially powerful framework to those seeking to develop practice in order to address palliative care needs of patients across different care settings, specialist fields, and within specialist palliative care itself. In short, developing palliative care practice dovetails with the strong emphasis reflected in the action research principles outlined in this chapter, namely: participation; engaging with different sets of values and beliefs; and generating knowledge and cultural change. However, there are also particular challenges for the action researcher in palliative care development, which by the very nature and constraints of palliative care practice, is complex.

References

Argyris, C. (1995) Participatory Action Research and Action Science Compared: A Commentary. *Journal of Managerial Psychology*, **10**: 20–26.

Argyris, C. (2006) *Reasons and Rationalizations: The Limits of Organzsational Knowledge*. Oxford: Oxford University Press.

Arieli, D., Friedman, V.J., and Agbaria, K. (2009) The Paradox of Participation in Action Research. *Action Research*, 7: 263–90.

Bradbury, H. and Reason, P. (2003) Action Research. *Qualitative Social Work*, 2: 155.

Chandler, D. and Torbert, B. (2003) Transforming Inquiry and Action. *Action Research*, 1: 133–52.

Coghlan, D. (2008) Authenticity as First Person Practice. *Action Research*, 6: 351–66.

Coghlan, D. and Brannick, T. (2010) *Doing Action Research in Your Own Organization*, 3rd edn. London: Sage.

Coghlan, D. and Casey, M. (2001) Action Research From the Inside: Issues and Challenges in Doing Action Research in Your Own Hospital. *Journal of Advanced Nursing*, 35: 674–82.

Gott, M., Seymour, J., Ingleton C., Gardiner, C., and Bellamy, G. (2012) 'That's Part of Everybody's Job': The Perspectives of Health Care Staff in England and New Zealand on the Meaning and Remit of Palliative Care. *Palliative Medicine*, 26(3): 232–41.

Gustavsen, B. (2003a) Action Research and the Problem of the Single Case. *Concepts and Transformation*, **8**: 93–9.

Gustavsen, B. (2003b) New Forms of Knowledge Production and the Role of Action Research. *Action Research*, **1**: 153–64.

Heron, J. (1996) *Co-operative Inquiry: Research into the Human Condition*. London: Sage.

Heron, J. and Reason, P. (2001) The Practice of Co-operative Inquiry: Research 'With' Rather Than 'On' People. In: P. Reason and H. Bradbury (eds), *Handbook of Action Research*, pp. 144–54. London: Sage.

Hockley, J. and Froggatt, K. (2006) The Development of Palliative Care Knowledge in Care Homes for Older People: The Place of Action Research. *Palliative Medicine*, 20: 835–43.

Marshall, J. (2004) Living Systemic Thinking. *Action Research*, 2: 305–25.

Marshall, J. (2006) Self-reflective Inquiry Practices. In: P. Reason and H. Bradbury (eds), *Handbook of Action Research*, pp. 335–42. London: Sage.

Marshall, J. and Reason, P. (2007) Quality in Research as 'Taking an Attitude of Inquiry'. *Management Research News*, 30: 368–80.

Munn-Giddings, C., McVicar, A., and Smith, L. (2008) Systematic Review of the Uptake and Design of Action Research in Published Nursing Research, 2000–2005. *Journal of Research in Nursing*, **13**: 464–77.

Ospina, S., Dodge, J., Godsoe, B., Minieri, J., Reza, S., and Schall, E. (2004) From Consent to Mutual Inquiry. *Action Research*, 2: 47–69.

Randall, F. and Downie, R.S. (2006) *The Philosophy of Palliative Care: Critique and Reconstruction*. Oxford: Oxford University Press.

Reason, P. (2003) Action Research and the Single Case: A Response to Bjorn Gustavsen and Davydd Greenwood. *Concepts and Transformation*, 8: 281–94.

Reason, P. (2006) Choice and Quality in Action Research Practice. *Journal of Management Inquiry*, 15: 187–203.

Reason, P. and Bradbury, H. (2006) Preface. In: P. Reason and H. Bradbury (eds), *Handbook of Action Research. Concise Paperback Edition*, pp. xxvi–xxxii. London: Sage.

Reason, P. and Bradbury, H. (2008a) Introduction. In: P. Reason and H. Bradbury (eds), *The Sage Handbook of Action Research: Participative Inquiry and Practice*, 2nd edn, pp. 1–10. London: Sage.

Reason, P. and Bradbury, H. (2008b) *The Sage Handbook of Action Research: Participative Inquiry and Practice*. London: Sage.

Reason, P. and Torbert, W.R. (2001) The Action Turn: Toward a Transformational Social Science. *Concepts and Transformation*, **6**: 1–37.

Sepúlveda, C., Marlin, A., Yoshida, T., and Ullrich, A. (2002) Palliative Care—the World Health Organization's Global Perspective. *Journal of Pain and Symptom Management*, 24: 91–6.

Shani, A.B. and Passmore, W.A. (1985) Organization Inquiry: Towards a New Model of the Action Research Process. In: D.D. Warrick (ed.), *Contemporary Organization Development: Current Thinking and Applications*, pp, 438–8. Glenview IL: Scott Foresman.

Torbert, W.R. (1999) The Distinctive Questions Developmental Action Inquiry Asks. *Management Learning*, **30**: 189–206

Waterman, H.A., Tillen, D., Dickson, R., and De Koning, K. (2001) Action Research: A Systematic Review and Assessment for Guidance. *Health Technology Assessment*, 5: 1–166.

Whitehead, J. and McNiff, J. (2006) *Action Research: Living Theory*. London: Sage.

Wicks, P.G., Reason, P., and Bradbury, H. (2008) Living Inquiry: Personal, Political and Philosophical Groundings for Action Research Practice. In: P. Reason and H. Bradbury (eds), *The Sage Handbook of Action Research: Participative Inquiry and Practice*, 2nd edn, pp. 15–30. Sage: London.

Wicks, P.G. and Reason, P. (2009) Initiating Action Research. *Action Research*, 7: 243–62.

Chapter 6

Appreciative inquiry

Caroline Nicholson and Julie Barnes

Introduction

'You matter because you are you. You matter to the last moment of your life, and we will do all we can not only to help you die peacefully but to live until you die' (Clark, 2002).

This famous quote from Dame Cecily Saunders, founder of the modern day hospice movement, links well to the three human universals espoused by David Cooperrider, co-founder of appreciative inquiry (AI). He posits that all human beings desire to have a voice, wish to be seen as essential to the group, and to be viewed as unique and exceptional. Thus, at the heart of both AI and palliative care are the shared fundamentals of relationship, collaboration, and unconditional positive regard.

This chapter sets out the philosophy and practices of AI as related to participatory research and palliative care. We draw on examples of our own involvement within AI in palliative care to illustrate the practices. We are mindful of the need to be informative and accessible and we hope to compel the reader to think and act on this chapter. Therein lies the tension: for, in aiming for clarity we do not wish to convey that AI is a method or recipe for 'doing' research; rather, we argue for AI as a choiceful way of thinking and practicing founded on core principles. To that end we cite Schwandt (2000: 320) who suggests: 'The work is not to choose which interpretative label; constructionist, hermeneutic, or something other best suits (your research methodology) but rather to confront the choices about how each of us wants to live the life of a social enquirer.' Living as an appreciative inquirer is particularly pertinent to palliative care, allowing for an engagement of both hearts and minds in the search for life in the situations and systems in and through which we find ourselves living and dying.

Appreciative inquiry: treasuring the questions

Devised in the USA by Cooperrider and Srivastva (1987) as a complement to conventional forms of action research, AI is an approach, method, and philosophy for promoting positive personal or organizational change and development. Appreciative inquiry seeks to discover and connect to those things that 'give life' to people, organizations, and human systems when they are most alive, effective, and healthy. It is founded on the assumption that inquiry into, and conversation about, strengths, successes, values, hopes, and dreams, triggers life-affirming change, and that 'human systems grow in the direction of what they persistently ask questions about'

(Cooperrider and Whitney, 1999: 248). It assumes that in every situation or organization something works well, and change can be leveraged through discovering, sustaining, and spreading these moments of excellence within the wider system.

Widely used in public and corporate institutions to develop organizations, the central tenet within AI is that in order to understand a person or situation (necessary for change and development) one needs to appreciate and openly inquire. Thus, at the centre of AI participatory research is a subtle but fundamental shift from 'analysis' (determining why something is like it is) to 'inquiry' (questioning to understand another person's view and thus seeing new perspectives and possibilities within a situation). This open discovery gains new knowledge through focusing on collaboration and personal narrative. Knowledge is sought and acquired in relationship with others and this increases the quality of the outcome. Whilst these processes are arguably found in all participatory research approaches, AI praxis is at its core, an intentional search for what gives life within an organization. By the asking of unconditional positive questions and the telling of stories to illuminate and understand organizations or individuals being at their best, the positive potential of the system is enhanced. This principle focus attends to what people value, and what is life-giving and sustaining within an organization. Only then are stories collectively discussed and analysed in order to create new, generative ideas or images that aid the desired developmental change. Cooperrider and Whitney write: 'AI is more than a method, it is a way of being with and directly participating in the life of a human system in a way that compels one to inquire into the deeper life-generating essentials and potentials of organizational existence' (Cooperrider and Whitney, 2001: 15). This we suggest is both an invitation and challenge to palliative care practitioners and researchers. Our experience suggests this approach helps us to reclaim the fundamental relatedness of palliative care practice which some argue has been lost in the increasing specialization and emphasis on problem-based symptom management in palliative care (Randall and Downie, 2006).

Core principles of appreciative inquiry

Whilst there is considerable variation in the way that AI is implemented, core principles underpin all these practices. Five original principles were identified and described as the DNA building blocks, the essential ingredient of AI (Watkins and Mohr, 2011). However, in keeping with the dynamic and collaborative endeavour of AI, these have been refined and expanded by AI practitioners over time. Hence, the principles are perhaps more aptly described as parameters, to be regarded as flexible underpinning and supporting to AI practice, rather than a rigid adherence to a rule or a code. We now consider the five initial principles alongside a sixth (wholeness) as principles particularly relevant to inquiry within the realm of palliative care.

The constructionist principle

The constructionist principle suggests that reality/ies is/are essentially constructed through social relationships and meaning making, and changes are co-created and ongoing. Based on social constructionism (Gergen and Gergen, 2003), this principle acknowledges the power and use of language in determining 'what we know' and 'how we know'. The language we use to describe ourselves and our experiences shapes our view of the world. This principle is foundational in that it not only allows inquirers to begin to understand a situation, but also to use words to activate change. Our experiences are always created and thus there is always the possibility of looking in on ourselves, taking an alternative view and creating something different. This perspective is perhaps challenging in situations of palliative care where an individual may feel powerless against a body that is declining, a welfare system that creates gateways to receiving good care, and a culture where people may shun contact with the dying for fear of their own mortality. However, living out the constructionist principle in AI practice allows for development and change, even a change in perspective, which then alters experience and reality. The following is an extract from an AI practitioner, recounting being with his partner, dying from breast cancer:

> I had the gift of accompanying my beloved during the last one and three quarter years and yesterday morning holding her hands, after a long breathing time she took a last deep breath and passed away for her last journey. Two minutes before I asked her, 'do you hear the church bell ring?' They started to ring for the 11 am church service nearby. I remember what I answered when Caroline asked me, 'What do you value the most despite the pain and sorrow?' and I said the best of it all is that I sense such a deep and intensive love for her, sometimes it's deeper than ever before which I didn't know I was capable of. . . . A great experience for me, to sense it—not just knowing it.
>
> (AI practitioner)

Poetic

The poetic principle develops the constructionist principle further, suggesting that human systems are not fixed and predictable, but rather living with past, present, and future realities. Stories are compelling and fundamental in revealing and creating our existence. Storytelling gathers information about feelings and experience, as well as facts. Like poetry, stories can be retold, creating metaphors and images of organizational or personal life. 'We can choose what we study and what we choose to study makes a difference. It describes—even creates—the world as we know it' (Whitney and Trosten-Bloom, 2003: 54). Within appreciative inquiry there is a deliberate focus on the *desired* story or image (understanding what we want more of), so that our inquiry focuses and develops the capacity of an organization/individual rather than, albeit inadvertently, lessening it. We suggest this is challenging in our current political and welfare systems and the formal research world where the words joy, vision, and dream do not sit well with outcomes and evaluations. However, we do well to remember that the emphasis on patient experience in current NHS reforms results in part from a lack of understanding and appreciation of the things that matter to patients in the most trying of situations (Patterson *et al.*, 2011). The poetic principle challenges researchers to think about deliberately noticing and enhancing the stories that give life to a person, situation, or organization; often the small and unremarked on things.

Simultaneity

This principle is based on the notion that inquiry and change are not separate but simultaneous entities. Watkins and Mohr (2011: 73) write: 'Inquiry is change!

The seeds of change are embedded in the first questions we ask.' Thus, the first questions we ask as appreciative inquirers are fateful to the inquiry and set the stage for what is discovered. The simultaneous nature of inquiry and change is a powerful feature of appreciative inquiry. It is exemplified in this account when working with the East Midland Dementia Group to create a regional response to the UK National Strategy 'Living with Dementia' (Barnes and Guild, 2011):

> When we asked participants for stories of what 'living well with dementia means to them', they raised their eyebrows in surprise. For people living with dementia and their carers, this is an unusual and challenging question—to even contemplate living well with a condition as disabling and distressing as dementia is a huge leap. As we explored this together, it became a question which people really enjoyed asking and answering. Together we learned about what people with dementia and their carers wanted for whole services and for local action plans. Individuals in our core group noticed the impact on themselves: they grew in confidence and felt empowered to speak out as their voices were valued and listened to by professionals. Partnerships developed and several of our original core group still contribute to local service planning forums and practitioner training.
>
> (Barnes and Guild, 2011)

This principle challenges linear models of change based on acquisition of knowledge, evaluation, recommendations, and subsequent change. It is more complex and chaotic to study and report findings when accounting for iterative and co-dependent change and inquiry. Van de Harr and Hosking (2004) argue that end point/product evaluation is inconsistent with relational approaches to research such as AI; rather relational research calls for relational and processual evaluation. Evaluation is local-historically constructed, that is, what locals think are the issues and what emerges for the interactions and relationships between participants and fellow workers. Crucially such evaluation is not separate from the process of AI data generation, but rather inherent within practice.

Anticipatory

'A vivid imagination compels the whole body to obey it' (Aristotle, cited in Cooperrider and Whitney, 1999: 258).

The anticipatory principle flows from the principle of simultaneity; and posits that the images we hold of our future inspire action. It argues for a choiceful engagement of future vision, for organizations and people move in the direction of the images they persistently hold. Within appreciative inquiry the collective imagination and stories of the future are perhaps the most important resources for generating constructive change. Whilst it is tempting to suggest future realities are difficult to engage with in palliative care, de Montaigne reminds us: 'To practice death is to practice freedom, a man who has learned how to die has unlearned how to be a slave' (de Montaigne, 1991: 95). Thus, the freedom to look at the future and craft our choices, albeit within bodily limitations, is possible only when we acknowledge that we will all die. At an organizational level, Allan Kelleher's Heath Promoting Palliative Care (Kellehear, 1999) argues that palliative care could be a collaborative social enterprise in which society, as well as individuals, must be supported to identify and direct their own informational and educational needs, and be provided with the opportunity to discuss death and dying issues important to them. The emphasis is on a participatory process—self-directed learning with support from palliative care workers.

It is not about 'denying' that death is a serious prospect for those under palliative care but rather recognition that the prospect of death is shared by all of us all of the time too (Kellehear, 1999: 79).

These are important foundations within inquiry in palliative care and demands of us as researchers to think about and be mindful of our own vision for the organization and people we inquire with.

Positivity

This principle contends that the more positive the images or questions to which a system is subject, the more positive and longer lasting the change. The principle draws on social and positive psychology such as Barbara Fredrickson's (2001) research on positive emotions which demonstrates that for a person to thrive and build their capacity, they require a ratio of three positive experiences to one negative. The Pygmalion or positive effect demonstrates that human systems have an observable tendency to evolve in the direction of those positive images that are the brightest and boldest, most illuminating, and promising. This so called heliotropic principle is used collectively within AI practice to create a positive vision of the future: 'We find that the more positive the question we ask, the more long-lasting and successful the change effort' (Cooperrider and Whitney, 1987: 258). The positive principle has been the subject of debate, with some AI practitioners suggesting it can create superficial, unchallenging conversations and that generativity is a more apt term (Bushe and Kassam, 2005).

However, the underlying principle emphasizes the importance of momentum and harnessing of hearts and minds to sustain it. Attention moves away from the binary of good or bad experiences to a movement forward; a growth perhaps that allows for the possibility of generative questions even in the most difficult of circumstances. It is perhaps the antithesis of simplistic happy talk to a risky, generous listening, and an intention towards life enhancing activity. The following extract exemplifies how a funeral celebrant and AI practitioner used this principle in her work:

> We are co-creating a funeral service which holds central the person who has died; and which fits with the family beliefs about life and death; and with their personal wishes for saying farewell. Working with cherished stories, memories, music, and poetry, we make this a unique ceremony and everyone is encouraged to participate in the way they wish. The focus is positive, although we do not shy away from talking about the difficult times too, finding ways to honour the whole person and their life achievements, events, and adventures. To hear that he or she (the deceased) 'would have loved what we did today' captures the essence of our intention and confirms my belief that creating a positive memorial and farewell through appreciative storytelling and co-creation is a healing process in itself.
>
> (Personal communication with Julie Barnes)

Wholeness

The wholeness principle stands on systems theory and argues for the importance and greater potential of the whole system in development and change (Bailey, 1994).

This incorporates wholeness in organizations and for individuals. Organizational wholeness seeks to engage stakeholders and think creatively about who these people might be. 'The whole must go in pursuit of itself; there is no other way to learn who they are' (Wheatley, 2006: 166). Important in this principle is the idea that inquiry can start anywhere in the system; and the inquiry will have an impact. Thus, often AI practitioners will ask participants to reflect on the first small changes that they can make. It is not that smallness denigrates the value of the work, rather that small changes can be owned at all levels of a system. Small changes can give time for current practices and support processes to develop and sustain change. This engagement with small changes seems particularly relevant within palliative care inquiry.

Individual wholeness works holistically to facilitate the integration of the different aspects of a person that can be split by the services we offer, and the psychological and social ways we manage and organize dying. Holding the whole person is a fundamental principle in palliative care. In their book *Healing Conversations*, Chadbourne and Silbert (2011) have written movingly about their experiences of using appreciative storytelling within their own families and particularly with dying relatives. They describe the powerful impact in: reconnecting and reconciling families; mending and enhancing relationships; and, easing conversations about life, death, and dying.

Appreciative inquiry processes

The practice of AI varies, dependent upon the unique situation of each inquiry. However, these practices are grounded in the principles detailed above, and in core processes. The key process within AI is asking unconditional positive questions to produce stories of organizations or individuals being at their best. This focuses attention on what people value, and therefore what is life giving and sustaining within an organization. These stories are collectively discussed in order to generate new ideas, understanding, and images that create the desired developmental change. This systematic process is often conceptualized as an AI cycle (see Figure 6.1), where each phase of the process is a discrete step, although the process is non-linear, overlapping, and on-going. The AI cycle can be as rapid and informal as a conversation but the process is often formalized as an organizational-wide process (or summit) involving every stakeholder working together. Typically AI summits work intensely over a period of 2–5 days to create high-level engagement, speedy organizational change and allow for the necessary engagement and participation to sustain change.

The 'definition' and 'discovery' phases aim at choosing a topic and utilizing stories to discover the positive capacity already existing within the organization. The 'dream' phase uses insight from the discovery phase to envision how the organization could change. Stories collected within the discovery phase are thematically presented and the participants generalize these into what the future would be like if there were more of these successful examples. Often this 'dream' is presented as a series of competing statements of strategic intent, for example, 'Having dementia is not a death sentence but the start of a new chapter in our life—if only more help was readily available to cope we could all be better prepared' (Barnes and Guild, 2011).

The 'design' phase focuses on the architecture of the organization and what needs to be in place for the dreams to be realized. This makes explicit the desired structures and

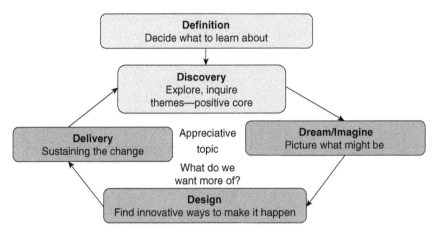

Fig. 6.1 Using appreciative inquiry—five 'D' cycle.

processes of the organization and actively seeks to include the wider system. The 'delivery' phase furthers this by examining specific innovations as well as what is necessary to sustain and celebrate collaborative and new ways of working. The cycle offers the opportunity for review and evaluation at any stage.

An exemplar of using the AI process is found in *Living Well with Dementia* (Barnes and Guild, 2011). The inquiry began with 'discovery' meetings with small groups of people with dementia and their carers. Together people explored what 'living well' meant to them and created images of a future in which everyone would be experiencing this, supported by caring, responsive services. Stories were gathered from a wide network and brought to a summit meeting of 180 people from many parts of the system, for example practitioners, managers, commissioners, third sector groups, and politicians. At this meeting further 'discovery' conversations were followed by collective 'dreaming' to create shared visions of what living well with dementia would look like. These informed a series of planning workshops in five local council areas following a process of 'design' and local action planning. People with dementia and their carers contributed to all these meetings. In a final summit of 320 people, we reviewed and celebrated the progress of the region and created a quality charter for dementia services in the East Midlands.

The process and outcomes of AI can be facilitated in other ways within palliative care research. Appreciative inquiry was chosen as the method of working with care providers (primary care staff and care home staff) to develop and sustain good end-of-life care for people with dementia living in residential care homes (Goodman *et al.*, 2012). Appreciative inquiry's stance and collaborative practices were considered of value in a setting which is often perceived as isolated and under-performing. It was recognized that participants (general practitioners, district nurses, and care home staff) were constrained by being based in different locations with limited resources to give additional time to meeting and working together. As it was not possible to engage with all people involved in providing and receiving care, the AI process was modified.

Short facilitative meetings were developed, and delivered over time within the care homes. This concentrated activity over six months was combined with ongoing support from the researchers. The method needed to be flexible to work with changing participant membership at the facilitated meetings, creating a team in the moment. The three main topics covered were: Meeting 1: 'an appreciation of practice through sharing stories'; Meeting 2: 'the development of practice through collective reflection on real time cases and development of interventions'; Meeting 3: 'sustaining the changes through participant led ideas of how to embed and expand their collaborative practices'.

Conclusion

In writing this chapter we are mindful not to present appreciative inquiry as a panacea for all ills, nor to set it in opposition to other participatory research methods. Moreover, whilst AI inquirers have shown evidence of change in healthcare systems, it would be naive to suggest that these outcomes were independent of power relations, engagement of key stakeholders and the finance to resource their spread and sustainability. However, we do suggest that the collaborative and generative nature of appreciative inquiry is powerful in helping specialist palliative care move beyond the often privileged and powerful positioning of some as 'experts' and others as 'recipients of knowledge/care', to a place where we are all co-learners and contributors. Weisbord writes: 'If I could ask one thing of a crystal ball in any situation it would not be what's wrong and how can we fix it, but what's possible here and who cares?' (Weisbord, 1987: 257). We would argue that within our dominant ideologies such questions are sufficiently challenging to require a set of parameters to help reframe our thinking.

In Einstein's words, 'No problem can be solved from the same level of consciousness that created it. We must learn to see the world anew' (cited in Bercher, 1979: 217). Appreciative inquiry, we suggest, allows us to see the world anew and to seek life and richness even in the context of death and dying. This is a powerful claim but one that we hope speaks through the stories interwoven through this chapter. For whilst we seek to extend our years, we are all mortal; and to return to Dame Cecily Saunders, dying contains gifts as well as tremendous challenges.

References

Bailey, K.D. (1994) *Sociology and the New Systems Theory: Toward a Theoretical Synthesis.* New York: State of New York Press.

Barnes, J. and Guild, J. (2011) Case Story: Living Well with Dementia: Creating a Regional Strategy for the East Midlands. In: J.M. Watkins, Mohr and Kelly. (eds), *Appreciative Inquiry: Change at the Speed of Imagination,* 2nd edn. San Francisco, London: Jossey Bass.

Bercher, K. (1979) Albert Einstein: 14 March 1879–18 April 1955 A Guide for the Perplexed. *Nature,* **278**: 215–18.

Bushe, G.R. and Kassam, A.F. (2005) When is Appreciative Inquiry Transformational? A Meta-Case Analysis. *Journal of Applied Behavioral Science,* 41: 161–81.

Chadbourne, J. and Silbert, T. (2011) *Healing Conversations Now, Enhance Relationships with Elders and Dying Loved Ones.* Ohio: Taos Institute Publications.

Clark, D. (2002) *Cicely Saunders—Founder of the Hospice Movement. Selected Letters 1959–1999.* Oxford: Oxford University Press.

Cooperrider, D.L. and Srivastva, S. (1987) Appreciative Inquiry in Organizational Life. *Research in Organizational Change and Development,* 1: 129–69.

Cooperrider, D.L. and Whitney, D. (1999) *Appreciative Inquiry: Collaborating for Change,* San Francisco: Barrett-Koehler.

Cooperrider, D.L. and Whitney, D. (2001) A Positive Revolution in Change: Appreciative Inquiry. *Public Administration and Public Policy,* 87: 611–30.

De Montaigne, M. (1991) *The Essays of Michel de Montaigne.* London: Allen Lane.

Fredrickson, B.L. (2001) The Role of Positive Emotions in Positive Psychology. *American Psychologist,* 56 (3): 218–26.

Gergen, M. and Gergen, K.J. (2003) *Social Construction: A Reader.* London: Sage.

Goodman, C., Amador, S., Mathie, E., Machen, I., Nicholson, C., King, D., and Baron, N.L. (2012) Evidence-based Interventions in Dementia: Changing practice in dementia care in the community: developing and testing interventions from early recognition to end of life: the final report of the Evidem end of life study. Final report to the NIHR Programme Grants for Applied Research.

Kellehear, A. (1999) Health-promoting palliative care: developing a social model for practice. *Mortality,* **4**: 75–82.

Patterson, M., Nolan, M., and Musson, G. (2011) From Metrics to Meaning: Culture Change and Quality of Acute Hospital Care for Older People. In: *Report for the National Institute for Health Research Service Delivery and Organization Programme.* HSMO: London.

Randall, F. and Downie, R.S. (2006) *The Philosophy of Palliative Care: Critique and Reconstruction.* Oxford University Press: USA.

Schwandt, T.A. (2000) *Three Epistemological Stances for Qualitative Inquiry: Interpretivism, Hermeneutics and Social Constructionism.* Thousand Oaks (CA): Sage.

Van de Harr, D. and Hosking D.M. (2004) Evaluating Appreciative Inquiry: A Relational Constructionist Perspective. *Human Relations,* 57: 1017.

Watkins, J.M., Mohr, B., and Kelly, R. (2011) *Appreciative Inquiry: Change at the Speed of Imagination,* 2nd edn. San Francisco: Pfeiffer/Wiley.

Weisbord, M.R. (1987) *Productive Workplaces Organizing and Managing for Dignity, Meaning, and Community.* San Francisco: Jossey-Bass.

Wheatley, M.J. (2006) *Leadership and the New Science: Discovering Order in a Chaotic World,* 3rd edn. San Francisco, CA: Berrett-Koehler Publishers.

Whitney, D. and Trosten-Bloom, A. (2003) *The Power of Appreciative Inquiry: A Practical Guide to Positive Change.* San Francisco: Berrett-Koehler Publishers Inc.

Section 2

Exemplars

Chapter 7

Community palliative care in Switzerland: from assessment to action

Steffen Eychmüller and
Franzisca Domeisen Benedetti

Introduction

As in many countries, most people suffering from advanced illness and facing death in Switzerland prefer to stay at home, or in their individually chosen surrounding for as long as possible, but factors influencing this decision can change over time (Munday et al., 2009). Increasingly, socio-economic factors will impact on this decision (Morrisson and Meier, 2004) and it is for such reasons that community palliative care has become a priority in end-of-life care in some countries (Department of Health, 2008; Gold Standards Framework, 2005).

There are several barriers to a more community-based healthcare system, and specifically for community palliative care in Switzerland. Whereas Switzerland provides free public hospital care for all (health coverage law), and healthcare reimbursement for outpatient medical services, costs for home care are paid largely by individuals themselves (out-of-pocket payment) and direct funding from local public money. Switzerland is a world leader in out-of-pocket payment per person, that is, the population pays more than 30% out-of-pocket payments, especially for dental medicine, home care, and residential aged care facilities (RACFs) (Lundy and Finder, 2009). In contrast to expressed wishes, around 80% of deaths occur within institutions (half in hospitals, half in RACFs), but not at home (Swiss Federal Office of Health, 2011). At present, almost all of the population has access to health insurance that covers primary healthcare, specialist medical services, and emergency and acute care in hospitals. This almost unlimited access to healthcare has led to rapidly increasing costs for medical insurance (which is compulsory for each person) and has come increasingly under pressure by politicians and the media. An intense debate is now underway regarding the costs of healthcare, especially in the last phase of life. Switzerland spends around 60 billion Swiss francs in healthcare for a population of 7.5 million people, or 11.5% of the gross national product. This is second to the USA in healthcare expenditure worldwide. Due to this comprehensive healthcare provision, community healthcare is seen to be of little importance.

Nonetheless, direct healthcare regularly occurs in the community and end-of-life issues and palliative care should be part of community members' health and social well-being (Fook and Kellehear, 2010; Kellehear, 2005). Palliative care services in Switzerland are scattered throughout the country, with some regions providing palliative care networks reaching international standards, and others without any access to palliative care (Eychmüller *et al.*, 2008). North-eastern Switzerland, which has St. Gallen as the major city, is one of the better developed regions in terms of palliative care, with a palliative care network—including specialist home care teams—that has been in existence since 2001. Even in this favourable situation, community palliative care is still a long way from being standard care at the end of life. The numbers of patients being cared for by the specialist palliative home care team remain low and unchanged over recent years. Informal feedback sessions have highlighted the cause of this being due to a lack of information, a perception of low quality care, and fears of additional costs.

This chapter presents an account of a regional initiative undertaken in north-eastern Switzerland to develop community-based palliative care. Drawing upon the model derived from work in Kerala (National Rural Health Mission, 2011), the account presented here describes the processes undertaken and the outcomes of the project.

Background and aim

The Kerala (India) Neighbourhood Network in Palliative Care (KNNPC) (NRHM, 2011) was identified as an excellent example of a model for community palliative care that effectively addresses some of the difficulties experienced by people who wish to die at home, and their primary carers. Much of the KNNPC's success is attributed to the active role of volunteers who run the programme. Palliative care professionals provide interventions as required, but only in support of the work by volunteers.

The key principle of KNNPC utilized in this project was the activation of community members to act as volunteers in order to access highly educated professionals, and also to establish a 24-hour home care service driven and financed by the community itself. Through this, caring for people who suffer from chronic or terminal illness has become a regular and normal part of daily activities in the community, and for each citizen. Apart from their profession or daily role, people contribute to this specific service in a variety of ways, such as giving small amounts of money, educating other community members, raising awareness about how to care, or by delivering direct patient care. There seems to be consensus that the integration of palliative care in normal community life will feed back to each person in the community when they themselves have a need for a similar service (Bollini *et al.*, 2004; Kumar, 2007).

Volunteer involvement is an integral part of community palliative care in Kerala, India. Impressed by this concept, and being able to accommodate an Indian colleague from Kerala, for a period of three months in our service, the project 'Community Palliative Care and Integration of Volunteers' was started in 2007 with support from a local foundation (Braun Foundation, Liechtenstein). We were aware of the challenges that existed to transfer an Indian model to Switzerland, mainly because of the different healthcare systems. The aim of this action research project was therefore to actively integrate not only community healthcare professionals, but also volunteers and other lay carers in the project. This was the reason why a participatory action research approach was chosen.

A participatory community development project was initiated and divided retrospectively into three steps:

1. Initial evaluation of status quo—the current situation in terms of service delivery and coordination of palliative care.

2. Initiation of community round tables (a meeting of peers for discussion and exchanging of views)—engagement of the community.

3. Formulation of recommendations and concrete action plans—reflections to build up and sustain local networks of palliative care and to raise awareness for palliative care in the community.

The project structure occurred dynamically as each major action was followed by a reflection within the project group and with individuals involved in the communities (core group), with each step being based on the previous work and not predicted in advance.

The project structure

For the purpose of this action research project, we chose three project communities in our region for further investigation:

1. The city of St Gallen—urban socio-demographic profile and a population of around 73,000 (Fachstelle für Statistik Kanton St Gallen, 2010; Hutter and Gerber, 2010) (suburbs not included). St Gallen is a university city with big industrial companies where administrative institutions are predominant.

2. The region and municipality of Flawil—rural area and a population of 10,000 inhabitants with small industries and agriculture where small villages are predominant.

3. The Principality of Liechtenstein—mixture of urban and rural characteristics with a population of 30,000 inhabitants.

In addition to their socio-demographic characteristics, these communities were chosen because existing contacts with non-palliative care professionals showed sympathy and support for this project—defined as a 'friendly audience' in regard to change management principles (Evans, 1996).

In each project community, one local research assistant was appointed in order to take the role as initial change agent for further development. The intention was to hand over this position as soon as each community/region was willing to take over the role. There was no plan to maintain this function longer than two years, which was the length of time the project was funded for.

Step one: Initial evaluation of status quo

Initially, the care networks in each community/region were assessed by network analysis. Network analysis is a method of exploring structure and interaction (the quantity and quality of relations) within social networks (Trezzini, 1998; Wellmann and Berkowitz, 1988). Local key individuals representing various groups and backgrounds were identified using a snowball technique and after a pilot phase, interviews were

Table 7.1 Themes of structured questionnaire with some examples

Themes of questionnaire	Examples
Socio-demographics about interviewees and their organizations	
Network analysis	Each interviewee described a maximum of five important professional relationships:
	◆ Frequency of collaboration
	◆ Quality of collaboration (inclusive obstacles and gaps for high quality collaboration)
Assessment of voluntary work in organization/ institution	
Assessment social support	Family, relatives, friends, neighbours
Desirable local care network for seriously ill and dying patients	Description of a desirable care network
Assessment of own integration into the local care network	
Other aspects of collaboration	What is missing?
Paragraph for interviewees working in volunteer organizations	

undertaken using structured questionnaires (Jansen, 2006) (see Table 7.1). This was undertaken over a four-month period from June to September 2007.

Thirty-five interviews were conducted across the three sites (see Table 7.2), with interviewees from various local institutions and organizations (see Table 7.3). From these interviews 133 relations between individuals, organizations, and institutions were analysed using network analysis. Analysis of the questionnaires showed the following status quo of palliative care in the investigated communities.

A variety of services offering palliative care in the local context were identified. The interview participants identified the following people as the most important collaborators in the care for seriously ill and dying people at home: outpatient registered nurses, family physicians (general practitioners), the mobile outpatient palliative care team, and the local hospice groups. A close cooperation between these collaborators was considered to be necessary to improve the quality of life of patients and their

Table 7.2 Number of interviews in each community/region

Region	N
St Gallen	13
Flawil	9
Principality of Lichtenstein	13
Total	35

Table 7.3 Number of organizations/institutions interviewed

Organization/institution	Number
Home care adults, children, and families	8
Specialist palliative care team in the community	2
Hospice volunteer group	3
General physician (GP)	5
Lung league (fundraising group)	2
Cancer league (fundraising group)	2
Protestant parish church	1
Catholic parish church	3
Social services (hospital based)	2
Information centres for older people (KBA, Sensen, ProSenectute)	2
Caritas (care provider for older people)	2
Tumour-und Breast Center ZeTup St Gallen (treatment and research centre)	1
Care/nursing homes	1
Palliativnetz Ostschweiz (PNO) (umbrella organization for palliative care activity)	1
Total	**35**

families in the physical, psychosocial, and spiritual domains. In terms of the availability of care and support, various offers for the care of seriously ill and dying people at home were made, and by this further opportunities for individual support and care identified.

Issues to do with communication in general were mentioned as the main barrier for good cooperation and collaboration between the organizations. A common platform, with a regular exchange between all parties in place, was not found in any of the communities. The interviewees agreed that a well-functioning network needs good, effective communication and coordination in order to be able to take over responsibilities (Thomas, 2003) and to provide individual palliative care at home.

The role of volunteers

In the initial survey, special attention had been given to find out the extent to which volunteers were integrated in the care of seriously ill and dying people in the community (Table 7.1). The interviewees stated that voluntary work in palliative care still needed to be better integrated, first of all as a conceptual framework and finally within daily clinical practice. The role of volunteers in palliative care seemed to be limited to direct care of patients and relatives (bedside care). The terms of reference could possibly be extended to include more fields of activity for socially active persons (Münzel, 2004), such as promotion of the topic within the broad public and fundraising activities. All interviewees concluded that volunteers should be a regular part of the community palliative care team and that the integration of volunteers is highly desirable and reasonable.

Step two: Initiation of community round tables

In each project community, the findings of step one were presented during a round table meeting facilitated by the local research assistant and attended by all interviewees and key stakeholders in the communities/regions. A status report was provided as the starting point for various activities. Formative and summative evaluations of the participants' contributions (Froggatt and Hockley, 2011) were gathered using the 'world café method' (Brown and Isaacs, 2008). This method was chosen to ensure a process driven by participants and to avoid predetermined outcomes. Some outcomes are highlighted below.

Composition of a future core group

As a first action point, core group members were identified, comprising the main professionals and actors in each community directly involved in the care of seriously ill and dying patients. This process was again coordinated by the local research assistant. In establishing the core group, the researchers stepped back from being the coordinators of the future community activities and handed over the role to the local community. The core group then met regularly and organized meetings/conferences for the health professionals and the public within the community to raise awareness and to set an agenda for further activities, including the integration of local politicians and community leaders. This structure was regarded as pertinent in all three communities and would give access to the politcal structure of the community. Independently from each other, they each initiated a palliative care forum, thereby successfully implementeing a communication platform. In ancient Rome, the term 'forum' was defined as an open public space in the middle of a Roman city.

Step three: Formulation of recommendations and concrete action plans

This third step in the project helped to build up and sustain local networks of palliative care as action plans, a checklist, and recommendations for both professionals and volunteers were fomulated.

From local action plans to general recommendations and a cantonal palliative care concept.

The intention of the research group to compose a final report for the project sponsor (Braun-Foundation, Liechtenstein) led to the creation of a series of resources. The idea of creating a generally valuable set of recommendations emerged. As a result of the initial status report and the local action plans provided by the project communities alongside the various recordings and experiences alongside the change process, a handbook (user guide) was published in German in July 2009 (Eychmüller et al., 2009). This guide contains recommendations and a checklist about how to start and initiate a process with concrete steps on how to establish a community-based palliative care network. Its recommendations have also been integrated, in part, into the cantonal palliative care concept producd by the cantonal government. More than 300 handbooks were sold by October 2011.

Checklist for the implementation of palliative care principles in the community

The idea of this checklist was to provide step-by-step guidance to help with issues that arise when building up and sustaining networks of palliative care in the community. The findings of this research project correspond with the Gold Standard Framework (GSF) Primary Care Programme (Thomas, 2003). The GSF programme was developed in 2003 by Dr Keri Thomas, an experienced general practitioner with special interest in palliative care, for local primary care.

> The name 'Gold Standards Framework' developed following discussion as to what best care would look like for people nearing the end of life, the 'gold standard' of care, and what is required to achieve this. Since then, the word 'gold' has come to symbolise an aspiration to best care for these most important of people, and an affirmation that, despite the busy pace of life, many feel this very important work that should be prioritised above all others—it is a matter of life and death.
>
> (GSF, 2005)

As with our project developed by local participants, the GSF Programme describes seven key tasks for successful end-life care: communication, coordination, control of symptoms, continuity of care, continued learning, carer support, and care of the dying. They were deliberately formulated to support teams and networks in the communties. For the purpose of our project we supplemented the seven key tasks and adapted them to the local needs. The checklist then contained 11 elements and goals (Table 7.4).

Recommendations for building up and sustaining a core group

As mentioned in step two, core groups in the communities were established consisting of the main actors in each community who were directly involved in the care of seriously ill and dying patients. This core group plays a crucial role in raising awareness of the need for improved palliative care in the community, and its composition may determine future success. Once a core group is built, it has to be sustained. To give direction and support to communities, the following recommendations give guidance (Table 7.5).

Recommendations for the integration of volunteers

If volunteers are to be integrated into the provision of palliative care settings at home, the following issue needs to be considered: there are two different types of volunteer activity—direct and indirect care (Claxton-Oldfield and Claxton-Oldfield, 2008). In direct care, patient and family care volunteers are responsible for the emotional and social support. Volunteers commit their time and deal confidentially with information that is sometimes not reported to healthcare professionals. In indirect care, there are fields of activities beside the direct patient care such as organizing fund raising/collecting donations, public relations and information (organization of events, reports, etc.), or coordination of a core team. A clear understanding needs to be determined in integrating volunteers to establish which of these approaches are being used, in order to avoid confusion for the volunteers and professionals working with them.

Table 7.4 Eleven elements and goals of the checklist for community palliative care

1. People/organizations: All people and organizations involved in the care of a seriously ill or dying patient are identified.

2. Voluntary work: Volunteers are integrated.

3. Communication: The family and the major network partners have access to information about palliative care in the community and are informed about the situation of those affected. The exchange among organizations and individuals is designed efficiently.

4. Coordination: The cooperation is transparent. The individual players are coordinated.

5. Control of symptoms: Distressing symptoms, and psychosocial/spiritual suffering, are relieved by competent treatment/therapy/counselling.

6. Continuity of care: Those affected (including single people) have the possibility of support around the clock.

7. Support of relatives: Relatives feel secure and supported by the care team. Anxieties can be minimized and emergencies can be largely avoided.

8. Continuous learning: The support team provides ongoing training. It is an everyday-based learning.

9. Care in the dying phase: Patients and families are supported during the last days of life.

10. Anchoring political and financial support: Palliative care is an issue in the community, organizations need to be identified that can assume financial responsibility, for example the church or other provider organizations.

11. Informing the population: The population is informed about the offer of palliative care in the community.

Table 7.5 Action points for core groups

1. The function of the core group: Define members, tasks and responsibilities, decision making process.

2. Coordination: Find a person for coordination of the core group—possibly a volunteer.

3. The core group's corporate design: Create a name for the group. An example is 'Palliative Care Forum community of . . .'

4. Constitute the core group officially and communicate to all interested people.

5. Formulate goals and objectives.

6. Instruments to achieve the objectives: Establish tools and strategies to achieve the goals. For example awareness: an information session organized for the population or presence in the local press.

7. Integrate other network partners: For example political authority in the community, nursing homes, and other local institutions, sympathizers or friendly audience.

8. Create a stimulating atmosphere: A friendly atmosphere is needed to assure openness, flexibility, trust, communication, responsibility, mutual appreciation, and interest.

Key findings and impacts of the work

The goal of the study was to prepare communities for a change in terms of active participation in end-of-life care. With the Kerala model of neighbourhood network palliative care as a starting point for reflection and discussion, this action research project succeeded in bringing together professionals, and finally politicians, in various projects and activities to improve community palliative care in our region.

This is extraordinary since Switzerland lacks a tradition of networking between professional organizations and volunteers. This part of Switzerland may be a long way from Kerala geographically and in terms of the healthcare system, and has yet to achieve a similar high proportion of people dying at home; however, this study demonstrates that the proposed pathway of assessing and coordinating community activities for terminally ill people, by the active participation and a grass-roots approach, can serve as a model for changing behaviour. This is relevant to the establishment of community palliative care in other regions of Switzerland and in other parts of the world with similar structures and problems.

As a direct consequence of this project, the idea of an award for 'Palliative Care in the Community' was first announced in September 2008 to emphasize the importance of the care of seriously ill and dying people and their families in all communities. The cantonal government, the cantonal hospital (including the centre of palliative care), and the regional palliative care network supported the award and invited the community council leaders in the canton of St Gallen, as well as the local healthcare organizations and individuals, to participate. Twelve communities participated in the award. It finally helped to demonstrate clearly the will of the community to improve and strengthen needs-based services founded on the activities of its inhabitants, as we have learned from the Kerala KNNPC project (Kumara, 2007). Today it can be stated that community palliative care has been adopted as an innovative approach in various communities in our region with regular palliative care networks now in place.

Challenges and reflections

For researchers

Participatory action research needs open-minded researchers. The role of the researcher resembles a facilitator rather than an active controller of a pre-determined research pathway. In principal, action research reflects the essential of any research: maintaining the ability to respond flexibly to new findings or results and to choose directions other than the initial planning. Leadership has been another aspect within this project requiring special attention: bringing professionals and non-professionals together was one of the goals of this project. Within the framework of action research there was the opportunity to practice real partnership and even to hand over research responsibility to non-professionals.

For our country

Switzerland is very much based on communities being the centrepiece of societal thinking. Such an environment facilitates participatory action research projects with the aim to activate community self-governance and responsibility. It might even be argued that without fostering the participation of all community members and local organizations this project might never have had any impact. Therefore, participatory action research might be *the* appropriate research method to alter healthcare delivery most effectively for severly ill and dying patients, in local communities with a high level of autonomy and self-responsibility.

Conclusion

This chapter has outlined a participatory action research project that brought together professionals, volunteers, and community leaders, to develop a community palliative care programme across three areas in north-eastern Switzerland. The Kerala KNNPC project in India had inspired thoughts behind the project, but the final outcome and the participation of core community groups working within the project has helped develop and sustain a community service in a country not known for its volunteerism. This chapter also proposes that participatory action research could be considered a major research method when healthcare delivery for people in end-of-life care would benefit from transformation.

Acknowledgement

The authors would like to thank the experts who participated in this study. Special thanks to our colleagues Michaela Forster and Nicole Schneider. They supported this project as local research assistants and helped it to be a success in north-eastern Switzerland.

Many thanks also to Kumar Suresh and Shamsudeen Moideen from the Kerala Neighbourhood Network in Palliative Care (KNNPC) in Kerala, India for providing the inspiration behind this project, and to Anne Williams from Western Australian Centre for Cancer and Palliative Care in Perth for the final review and editing.

References

Bollini, P., Venkateswaran, C., and Suresh, K. (2004) Palliative Care in Kerala, India: A Model for Resource Poor Settings. *Onkologie*, **27**: 138–42.

Brown, J. and Isaacs, D. (2008) *The World Café: Shaping our Future through Conversations that Matter.* San Francisco: Berrett-Koehler Publishers.

Claxton-Oldfield, S. and Claxton-Oldfield, J. (2008) Keeping Hospice Palliative Care Volunteers on Board: Dealing with Issues of Attrition, Stress, and Retention. *Indian Journal of Palliative Care*, **14**(1): 30–37.

Department of Health (2008) *National End of Life Care Programme.* Available from: http://www.endoflifecare.nhs.uk/eolc/.

Evans, R. (1996) *The Human Side of School Change: Reform, Resistance, and the Real-Life Problems of Innovation.* San Francisco: Jossey-Bass Inc.

Eychmüller, S., Domeisen, F., Forster, M., and Schneider, N. (2009) *Palliative Care in Gemeinde: ein Handbuch zur Vernetzung. Erfahrungen aus einer Ostschweizer Studie.* St Gallen: Palliativzentrum St Gallen.

Eychmüller, S., Schmid, M., and Müller, M. (2008) *Palliative Care in der Schweiz: Nationale Bestandsaufnahme.* Available from: http://www.zhaw.ch/fileadmin/user_upload/engineering/_Institute_und_Zentren/IDP/forschungsschwerpunkte/DAS/reasearch_reports/bericht_pallcare_survey08.pdf.

Fachstelle für Statistik Kanton St Gallen (FfS-SG) (2010) *Fachstelle für Statistik Kanton St Gallen. Der Kanton St Gallen und seine Menschen in Zahlen.* St Gallen: Fachstelle für Statistik Kanton St Gallen (FfS-SG).

Fook, J. and Kellehear, A. (2010) Using Critical Reflection to Support Health Promotion Goals in Palliative Care. *Journal of Palliative Care,* **26**(4): 295–302.

Froggatt, K. and Hockley, J. (2011) Action Research in Palliative Care: Defining an Evaluation Methodology. *Palliative Medicine,* **25**(8): 782–87.

Gold Standards Framework (2005) *Gold Standards Framework.* Available from: http://www. goldstandardsframework.org.uk/about_GSF/Why Gold, download 25 February 2012.

Hutter, T. and Gerber, E. (2010) *Statistisches Jahrbuch der Stadt St.Gallen.* St Gallen: Fachstelle für Statistik Kanton St Gallen (FfS-SG).

Jansen, D. (2006) *Einführung in die Netzwerkanalyse—Grundlagen, Methoden, Forschungsbeispiele,* 3rd edn. Wiesbaden: VS Verlag für Sozialwissenschaften.

Kellehear, A. (2005) *Compassionate Cities: Public Health and End-of-Life Care.* London: Routledge.

Kumar, S. (2007) Kerala, India: A Regional Community-Based Palliative Care Model. *Journal of Pain and Symptom Management,* **33**(5): 623–7.

Lundy, J. and Finder, B.D. (2009) *Cost Sharing for Healthcare: France, Germany, and Switzerland.* Menlo Park, CA: The Henry J. Kaiser Family Foundation. Available from: http://www.kff.org/insurance/upload/7852.pdf.

Morrisson, R.S. and Meier, D.E. (2004) Palliative Care. *New England Journal of Medicine,* **350**: 2582–90.

Munday, D., Petrova, M., and Dale, J. (2009) Exploring Preferences for Place of Death with Terminally Ill Patients: Qualitative Study of Experiences of General Practitioners and Community Nurses in England. *British Medical Journal,* **338**(b2391).

Münzel, G., Guzzi Heeb, S., Kadishi, B., Nadai, E., and Schön-Bühlmann, J. (2004) *Sozialberichterstattung Schweiz. Bericht zur Freiwilligenarbeit in der Schweiz.* Neuchâtel: Bundesamt für Statistik.

National Rural Health Mission (2011) *National Rural Health Mission Palliative Care Project.* Available from: http://www.instituteofpalliativemedicine.org/.

Swiss Federal Office of Health (2011) *Palliative Care.* Available from: http://www.bag.admin. ch/themen/medizin/06082/index.html?lang=de.

Thomas, K. (2003) *Caring for the Dying at Home: Companions on the Journey.* Oxford: Radcliffe Medical Press Ltd.

Trezzini, B. (1998) Theoretische Aspekte der sozialwissenschaftlichen Netzwerkanalyse. *Schweizerische Zeitschrift für Soziologie,* **24**(3): 511–44.

Wellmann, B. and Berkowitz, S.D. (1988) *Social Structures: A Network Approach.* Cambridge: Cambridge University Press.

Chapter 8

Facilitating bereavement support for people with intellectual disabilities in England

Sue Read

The aim of this chapter is to share my journey of using action research where the practice setting incorporates one particular marginalized group, people with intellectual disabilities (ID). It will describe my progress from conducting research *on* people with intellectual disabilities to working alongside *with* people with intellectual disabilities, as part of the emancipatory element of participatory action research (PAR). Using examples of action research conducted over a 20-year period, in the area of bereavement and end-of-life care, I will demonstrate not only how action research can be used to change and improve practice, but also how it can be used to empower and change the researcher's stance around involving 'users' of services as co-researchers within the sensitive area of death, dying, and bereavement.

Initially, I will introduce and define the ID population and the inherent challenges when involving people with intellectual disabilities as 'users' of health services within the research process. The introduction of research examples will underpin the essential elements of PAR, and provide the foundation for personal reflections on the emergent challenges of effectively conducting this work with a distinctly marginalized and disempowered population.

Research and marginalized populations

As previous chapters have identified, action research provides a methodological framework that deliberately integrates theory into practice in a meaningful way, retaining a sustainable force for change amongst global healthcare settings (Williams *et al.*, 2011). Users of healthcare services can bring a rich range of personal skills, knowledge, experiences, and abilities that can contribute well to the research arena, complementing the expertise of the researcher (Royal College of Nursing, 2007), offering alternative perspectives, and ensuring that research priorities are realistic and appropriate (Steele, 2004).

People with ID are users of health and social care services and can make useful contributions to the research arena (Williams and England, 2005), yet because of the nature of their disabilities, involving them in research may be difficult. However, good research practices involve users and carers across all steps of the research continuum, and some research (e.g. practitioner research) conducted without such involvement could be seen as having 'major limitations when applied to practice' (Fox *et al.*, 2007: 146). Wright and Rowe (2005) advocate active and equitable collaboration as being crucial to service user involvement generally. Styles of research involvement include: consultation; collaboration; or user controlled (Consumers in National Health Service Research Group, 2001). Consultation involves researcher-led activities with passive consumer involvement (e.g. being consulted about the design process). Collaboration includes joint and equal partnership working where users and carers are responsible for the design and conduct of the research. User-controlled research proactively places the consumer as the driving force of the research (Fox *et al.*, 2007; Lowes and Hulatt, 2005) ultimately reducing the 'asymmetrical relationships' power status between scientific and experiential knowledge (Abma *et al.*, 2009).

Service user involvement in research 'has increasingly become a significant develop-ment on the research landscape' (McLaughlin, 2009: 1591); however, involving mar-ginalized groups within the research process can sometimes be difficult because it has not been done enough to be perceived as being easy (Read and Corcoran, 2009). The key challenges to active participation include the varied attitudes of researchers and professionals, resources, and values (Gilbert, 2004), so forward planning is required from the researchers involved.

Research remains a powerful and important 'finding out' tool that can send explicit messages to those who participate; by involving people in research suggests that all the participants have a contribution to make. It implies that participant contributions will be useful and meaningful and confirms how much researchers value the time, experi-ences, and contributions that participants have to offer (Read and Corcoran, 2009). Everyone has a story to tell, and people with ID often have simple, yet incredibly pow-erful tales about their lives and experiences (Atkinson *et al.*, 2000; Read and Bowler, 2007), and indeed views about their own impending death (Tuffrey-Wijne and Davies, 2003). Researchers working in this arena need to be proactive in finding ways of help-ing people with ID to communicate and share their experiences in different ways.

Understanding intellectual disability

The Department of Health (DH) in England describes people with a learning disability as 'having a reduced ability to understand new or complex information or to learn new skills (impaired intelligence) with a reduced ability to cope independently (impaired social functioning) which started before adulthood and with a lasting effect on development' (DH, 2001: 14). (The term learning disabilities is the current term within the UK; other terms include intellectual disabilities and mental retardation. From here on in, the term intellectual disabilities will be used throughout this chapter.) This means that some people with ID may find it harder than others to learn, understand, and communicate. Those with complex and multiple, associated disabili-ties will need full time support with their everyday living tasks (Read and Morris, 2009). Mencap (a United Kingdom (UK) charity, often described as 'the voice of peo-ple with a learning [sic] disability') estimate that there are 1.5 million people with ID in the UK (Mencap, 2011). However, they remain a marginalized, disadvantaged population particularly when it comes to palliative, end-of-life care and bereavement support.

With better healthcare generally, and better neonatal care specifically, this population is increasing at both ends of the spectrum (children and older people) and healthcare professionals can expect increasing contact and demands from this group (Emerson and Hatton, 2008; Parrot, *et al.*, 2008; RCN, 2011). One of the most common age-related illnesses is cancer and whilst there has been an increase of literature in recent years around end-of-life care and bereavement support for people with ID, there is limited research from the perspectives of people with ID themselves and particularly for those with severe and profound disabilities (Maaskant *et al.*, 2010).

Regardless of any clinical diagnosis or other label ascribed to people with ID, they remain distinct individuals, with different personalities, characteristics, preferences, needs, wants, and dreams, just like everyone else in today's contemporary society. Whilst people with ID vary tremendously in terms of their capabilities and associated needs, communication remains a fundamentally important issue. The challenges to both service providers and care deliverers alike is to identify the holistic needs of each individual in order to ensure that optimum quality of life is achieved, particularly when end of life is approaching.

'Intellectual disability research has an important role to play in identifying areas of need, areas of best practice, and informing evidence based practice' (Townsend, 2011: 114), and people with ID can constructively contribute to the research arena (Gibbs and Read, 2010). However, they may need tailored help to participate because of their varied needs. For example, within data analysis, the use of visual representations of data (i.e. bar graphs instead of numbers) have been found to be useful in breaking data down into manageable 'chunks'; also, collaborating with and helping people with ID themselves to identify effective questions around analysis, ensures transparency of research processes for the person with an ID (Kramer *et al.*, 2011).

The practitioner researcher's journey

The practitioner researcher is described by Robson (1997) as someone who holds down a job in a particular area whilst at the same time carries out a systematic enquiry which is of relevance to that job. Consequently 'practitioner researchers are people who are part of the world that they are researching in such a way that an academic researcher cannot be' (Reed and Proctor, 1995: 5). The primary aim of practitioner research is to improve practice (Reed and Procter, 1995). Much of my primary research has been concerned with impact on practice, and change innovation, with a particular focus on ID practice. Subsequently, practitioner action research, as a strand of action research seeking to overcome issues of oppression and marginalization (Kramer *et al.*, 2011; Williamson *et al.*, 2011), remains an ideal approach. Practitioner action research supports inclusive research, where people with an ID can be actively involved in the formulation of research problems, data collection, and analysis (Kramer *et al.*, 2011).

Much of my research interest lies in the sensitive area of death, dying, and bereavement with marginalized populations, specifically (but not exclusively) people with ID. A fundamental driver across all the examples of research introduced in this chapter is to address the lack of practice knowledge and resources available to support this population within caring environments.

The journey begins

As a neophyte researcher, the first serious piece of research I conducted was my PhD, completed in 2004 and entitled 'Bereavement counselling for people with an intellectual disability: Journeys without maps' (Read, 2004). The emotional needs of people with ID remain frequently neglected (Arthur, 2003), and this practitioner action research study which established a specialized bereavement counselling service for adults with intellectual disabilities, within a voluntary bereavement counselling agency, helped to address this issue. This study ultimately led to the development of a bereavement counselling manual (Read, 2007) to support counselling practice. As a clinician (i.e. ID nurse and latterly bereavement counsellor) and an academic, such combined skills helped me to conduct a research study that had practice at its heart. The research arose from practice, for the purpose of advancing practice and as such began as a practitioner-led enquiry (McLeod, 1999). As May (2001: 21) reminds us: 'It is both the experiences of the researched *and* researchers which are important' and this was reflected throughout the study.

Thus, the PhD research study developed out of a practitioner-led inquiry into a perceived gap in the service provision, namely bereavement counselling for people with ID. I always felt that action research chose the project, rather than a deliberate decision made by myself to use action research, since, at the time, there was no other similar study to replicate or learn from. Hence the title: 'Journeys without maps' as at times it felt that I was navigating through unchartered territory; the navigation system being the cyclical process of the action research framework can simultaneously be exciting and fearful.

The research began as a practitioner inquiry into the nature of the bereavement counselling offered to people with ID. In using practitioner action research, the symmetry between practice innovation and research was held in balance. Therefore, as the change agent, I had a pivotal role in both developing and maintaining the research. It was an approach that emphasized collaboration and participation, which in this instance had to be maintained over a significant period of time (six years). My relationship with the counselling practice area of ID remained a crucial element of the research and its subsequent development.

The research study evolved over a six-year period of time (see Figure 8.1), and was conducted in four discreet but interconnected phases. It was not envisaged at the beginning that the outcome would be a bereavement counselling manual. All four phases of the research study supported the emergent focus on the development of a counselling manual to support bereaved people with ID. Fundamental to this was the practitioner working within the action research framework.

Five research methods were used to explore the bereavement counselling experiences of people with ID and to assist in the identification of the core content and process of the manual. The five methods included: focus group discussions, a counselling session evaluation sheet, a self-rating questionnaire, biographies, and a pre- and

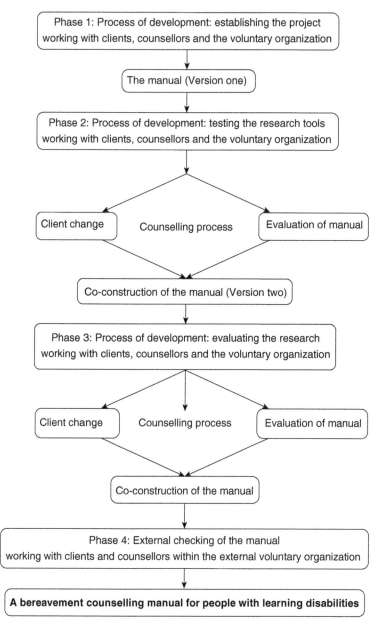

Fig. 8.1 An overview of the four phases of the participatory action research process.
Reproduced with permission from Sue Read, Bereavement counselling and support for people with learning disabilities: a manual to develop practice, Quay Books, London, Copyright © 2007.

post-bereavement counselling checklist. These methods were designed to help the researcher address the research questions in a rigorous and triangulated fashion (from a client, counsellor, and organizational perspective), during phases two and three of the study. Such triangulation of data collection methods (or mixed method designs) enabled me to: investigate different aspects of the same phenomena (Crawford and

Christenson, 1995); obtain a variety of information on the same issue; use the strengths of each method to overcome the deficiencies of the other; achieve a higher degree of validity and reliability; and, overcome the deficiencies of single-method studies (Sarantakos, 1998).

The PhD in essence provides research training, and I learned much about the action research process and associated challenges around relinquishing power and control over to others, to drive and shape the ultimate direction of the research. On reflection, this was probably one of the most difficult challenges of this first research experience. However, it taught me much about the importance of user and carer participation, collaboration, and active involvement, as well as the huge potential for more user controlled and user driven research, as opposed to the contributions of people with ID as solely passive research participants.

A further journey

Building on my research experiences, another action research project was undertaken that involved users (people with ID) and carers (nurses, parents, psychologists, doctors) to develop a series of leaflets and pamphlets around bereavement and end-of-life care support. I coordinated two groups of collaborators interested in developing accessible resources, which developed, refined, and shaped the content of the leaflets and booklets through the cyclical process of action research. With small pockets of local funding, three bereavement leaflets were developed and formally evaluated (Read and Spall, 2006). These addressed the holistic bereavement needs from the perspective of the person with ID, parents, and carers. The leaflets are now into their third edition and have been freely available since 2005.

Similarly, a participatory action research project was used to develop a series of six end-of-life care leaflets/booklets: four leaflets for people with ID; a booklet for personal carers; and a booklet for professional carers (see Figure 8.2). Working alongside people with ID, the clergy, parents and nurses, and psychologists (as well as consulting with advocacy groups), the leaflets and booklets were shaped and reshaped in terms of content and formats to ensure maxim accessibility. Such a holistic approach to care and support prior to and following death was seen as pivotal to the success of these resources.

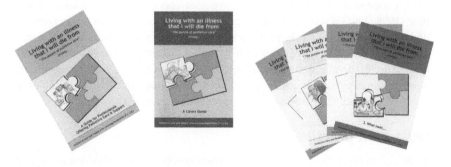

Fig. 8.2 Leaflets to support end-of-life care.
Reproduced with kind permission from Sue Read.

Subsequent funding has since been secured to work alongside two advocacy organizations in different parts of the country using participatory action research to collaboratively develop a resource for people with ID to use to support each other when experiencing loss. Whilst meeting and supporting people with ID is time consuming, it is crucial to developing resources that meet the needs of the very people who generated the ideas, ensuring they remain fit for purpose.

In a more recent participatory action research study to develop an interactive, web-based tool to support bereavement and loss (Read *et al.*, in press), people with ID were co-researchers on the project from a process and content perspective, shaping the development of the tool and influencing the methodology used within the refining processes. The outcome of this collaboration, working alongside people with an ID as co-researchers, has produced an accessible, flexible piece of software that can facilitate individual storytelling around loss and bereavement and promote spontaneous expression that can be shared with others. This is a clear example of collaborative research that places people with ID as joint equal partners, as opposed to passive recipients (Fox *et al.*, 2007; Lowes and Hulatt, 2005).

Reflections on the challenges

One of the strengths of participatory action research is the cyclical process of planning, implementing, evaluating, and feedback. This creates a strong relationship between theory and practice to create and clarify new meanings and understandings about the topic being investigated. Using a research design that is open and flexible and does justice to the complexities of the topic under investigation can be very cathartic and empowering, but can also be daunting for neophyte researchers. The more action research I have been involved in, the more confident I feel to work with the uncertainty and the apparent 'lack of control' within the research conducted. In my experience, action research provided the framework for developing reflective practice in which practitioners and researchers critically challenged assumptions about that practice, and ultimately steered practice innovation with the involvement of people with intellectual disabilities.

On reflection, people with ID should have been invited to participate in the steering group that managed the research in the first research example provided, since collaboration is seen as central to enable effective communication and to ensure maximum participation of all those involved. As a naive researcher this was overlooked, as at that time (1998–2004) it was not standard practice to be so inclusive. As I have grown to understand and appreciate the principles and potential of action research more clearly, and worked alongside with people with ID within this process, I have recognized the importance of their unique and valuable contributions. Over the years I have become more determined to involve this population across the research continuum, not just as passive participants, as evidenced in my more recent examples.

Impact on practice

These action research studies, developed from practice, were embedded in practice and produced products (a manual, booklet, electronic tool) that would ultimately feed back into practice. Such collaborative efforts, which systematically build clinician feedback into their development and dissemination will make the resources more effective, flexible, more dynamic, and more likely to be used (Addis *et al.*, 1999); and are the essence of action research (Carr and Kemmis, 1986; Grbich, 1999). The data generated and analysed throughout these projects provided a firm evidence base for the resources, ensuring that they remained firmly rooted in practice for this marginalized population. The manual (Read, 2007), although predominantly a resource to support counselling practice, also incorporates research tools and procedures (e.g. assessment formats, consent procedures); these helped to generate the data which in turn supported the manual content.

Conclusion

End-of-life care is a developing concept, and the 'movement to involve consumers in cancer research has grown rapidly since the early 1990s' (Stevens and Wilde, 2005: 109). Educators, practitioners, and researchers alike continue to strive to understand the patient's experience as s/he journeys toward death, in an effort to appreciate what is required at this difficult time (Read and Maslin-Prothero, 2011). Emphasis is placed on the implementation of consumer views in palliative care generally (NICE, 2004a; 2004b), and there is a developing interest in how this can be effectively achieved. The research examples provided in this chapter demonstrate well that action research has been an excellent tool to engage with people with ID, as well as a range of clinicians, practitioners, academics, volunteers, and parents, promoting empowerment and acting as the catalyst for the sharing of personal experiences. Whilst research can be a vehicle for listening and promoting meaningful consultations with people with an intellectual disability, participatory action research provided the methodological framework to ensure that this can happen, particularly with marginalized populations.

Bereavement counselling and support is a crucial element in end-of-life care as survivors seek to make sense of a world that is significantly different, with the heavy absence of a loved one's physical presence. For a person with an ID, who may struggle with complex concepts such as palliative care, dying, and death, accommodating the finality of this loss continues to be difficult. Participatory action research has provided a flexible framework to develop a range of resources to support individuals, parents, and professional carers, from a holistic perspective that has a firm practical orientation.

References

Abma, T.A., Nierse, C.J., and Widdershoven, A.M. (2009) Patients as Partners in Responsive Research: Methodological Notions for Collaborations in Mixed Research Terms. *Qualitative Health Research*, **19**: 401–15.

Addis, M.E., Wade, W.A., and Hatgis, C. (1999) Barriers to Dissemination of Evidenced Based Practices: Addressing Practitioners' Concerns about Manual-Based Psychotherapies. *Clinical Psychology: Science and Practice*, **6**(4): 430–41.

Arthur, A.R. (2003) The Emotional Lives of People with Learning Disability. *British Journal of Learning Disabilities*, **31**: 25–30.

Atkinson, D., McCarthy, M., Walmsley, J., *et al.* (2000) *Good Times, Bad Times: Women with Learning Difficulties Tell their Stories.* Kidderminster: British Institute of Learning Disabilities.

Carr, W. and Kemmis, S. (1986) *Becoming Critical: Education, Knowledge and Action Research.* London: The Falmer Press.

Crawford, H.J. and Christensen, I.B. (1995) *Developing Research Skills: A Laboratory Manual.* Boston: Alleyn & Bacon.

Consumers in National Health Service Research (2001) *Getting Involved in Research: A Guide for Consumers.* Eastleigh: Consumers in National Health Service Research.

Department of Health (2001) *Valuing People: A New Strategy for Learning Disability for the 21st Century.* London: Department of Health. Crown Copyright 2001.

Emerson, E. and Hatton, C. (2008) *Estimating Future Need for Adult Social Care Services for People with Learning Disabilities in England.* Lancaster: Institute for Health Research, Lancaster University.

Fox, M., Martin, P., and Green, G. (2007) *Doing Practitioner Research.* London: Sage.

Gibbs, M. and Read, S. (2010) Involving People with Intellectual Disabilities in Research: Participation and Emancipation. In: P.M. Roberts and H.M. Priest (eds), *Healthcare Research: A Handbook for Students and Practitioners*, pp. 247–55. London: John Wiley.

Gilbert, T. (2004) Involving people with learning disabilities in research: issues and possibilities. *Health and Social Care in the Community*, 12(4): 298–308.

Grbich, C. (1999) *Qualitative Research in Health; an Introduction.* London: Sage.

Kramer, J.M., Kramer, J.C., García, E., and Hammel, J. (2011) Following Through to the End: The Use of Inclusive Strategies to Analyse and Interpret Data in Participatory Action Research with Individuals with Intellectual Disabilities. *Journal of Applied Research in Intellectual Disabilities*, 24: 263–73.

Lowes, L. and Hulatt, I. (eds) (2005) *Involving service Users in Health and Social Care Research.* Oxfordshire: Routledge.

Maaskant, M., van de Kerkhof, R.M., van Bomme, H., and van de Wouw, W. (2010) How do Persons with Severe and Profound Intellectual Disabilities Experience their Approaching Death and How can they be Supported? In: V.P. Prasher (ed.), *Contemporary Issues in Intellectual Disabilities*, pp. 75–80. New York: Nova Science.

May, T. (2001) *Social Research: Issues, Methods and Process*, 3rd edn. Buckingham: Open University Press.

McLaughlin, H. (2009) Keeping Service User Involvement in Research Honest. *British Journal of Social Work*, 40: 1591–608.

McLeod, J. (1999) *Practitioner Research in Counselling.* London: Sage.

MENCAP: *The Voice of Learning Disability.* http://www.mencap.org.uk/all-about-learning-disability (accessed 15 October 2011).

National Institute for Health and Clinical Excellence (NICE) (2004a) *Improving Support and Palliative Care for Adults with Cancer.* London: National Institute for Health and Clinical Excellence.

National Institute for Health and Clinical Excellence (NICE) (2004b) *Support and Palliative Care Services for Adults with Cancer: Understanding NICE Guidance-Information for Adults with Cancer, their Families and Carers and the Public.* London: National Institute for Health and Clinical Excellence.

Parrott, R., Tilley, N., and Westenholme, J. (2008) Changing Demography and Demands for Services for People with Complex Needs and Profound and Multiple Learning Disabilities. *Tizard Learning Disability Review*, 13(3): 26–34.

Read, S. (2004) Bereavement Counselling for People with an Intellectual Disability: Journeys Without Maps. Unpublished thesis, Staffordshire: Keele University.

Read, S. (2007) *Bereavement Counselling and Support for People with Learning Disabilities: A Manual to Develop Practice*. London: Quay Books.

Read, S. and Bowler, C. (2007) Life Story Work and Bereavement: Shared Reflections on its Usefulness. *Learning Disability Practice*, **10**(4): 10–15.

Read, S. and Corcoran, P. (2009) Research: A Vehicle for Listening and Promoting Meaningful Consultation with People with an Intellectual Disability. *The British Psychological Society: Qualitative Methods in Psychology Section*, **8**: 29–37.

Read, S. and Maslin-Prothero, S. (2011) The Involvement of Users and Carers in Health and Social Research: The Realities of Inclusion and Engagement. *Qualitative Health Research*, **21**(5): 704–13.

Read, S. and Morris, H. (2009) *Living and Dying with Dignity, the Best Practice Guide for End of Life Care for People with Learning Disability*. London: MENCAP.

Reed, J. and Proctor, S. (eds) (1995) *Practitioner Research in Health Care: The Inside Story*. London: Chapman & Hall.

Read, S. and Spall, B. (2006) Bereavement and People with a Learning Disability: A Practice Initiative in Response to a Local Need. *Learning Disability Practice*, **9**(2): 8–15.

Read, S., Nte, S., and Corcoran, P. (in press) Web Based Bereavement Software for People with Intellectual Disabilities: Active Engagement for Effective Development. *Journal of Applied Research in Intellectual Disabilities*.

Robson, C. (1997) *Real World Research: A Resource for Social Scientists and Practitioner—Researchers*, 5th edn. Oxford: Blackwell.

Royal College of Nursing (2007) *User Involvement in Research by Nurses*. London: Royal College of Nursing.

Royal College of Nursing (2011) *Learning from the Past—Setting Out the Future: Developing Learning Disability Nursing in the Future*. London: Royal College of Nursing.

Sarantakos, S. (1998) *Social Research*, 2nd edn. Hampshire: Palgrave.

Steele, R. (ed.) (2004) *Involving the Public in NHS, Public Health and Social Care Research: Briefing Notes for Researchers*. Hampshire: Involve.

Stevens, T. and Wilde, D. (2005) Consumer Involvement in Cancer Research. In: L. Lowes, and I. Hulatt (eds), *Involving Service Users In Health And Social Care Research*, pp. 97–111. Oxfordshire: Routledge.

Townsend, C.E. (2011) Developing a Comprehensive Research Agenda for People with Intellectual Disability to Inform Policy Development and Reform. *Journal of Policy and Practice in Intellectual Disability*, **8**(2): 113–24.

Tuffrey-Wijne, I. and Davies, J. (2003) This is my Story: I've Got Cancer. 'The Veronica Project': An Ethnographic Study of Experiences of People with Learning Disabilities who have Cancer. *British Journal of Learning Disabilities*, **35**: 7–11.

Williams, V. and England, M. (2005) Supporting People with Learning Difficulties to do their Own Research. In: L. Lowes and I. Hulatt (eds), *Involving Service Users in Health and Social Care Research*, pp. 30–40. London: Routledge.

Williamson, GR., Bellman, L., and Webster, J. (2011) *Action Research in Nursing & Healthcare*. London: Sage.

Wright, C. and Rowe, N. (2005) Protecting Professional Identities Service User Involvement and Occupational Therapy. *British Journal of Occupational Therapy*, **68**(1): 45–7.

Chapter 9

Palliative interventions and acute respiratory care in Ireland

Patricia White and Marie Lynch

Introduction

This action research project focuses on the integration of palliative care for people with advanced respiratory disease. Whilst based in a respiratory department of a large urban acute hospital in Ireland, the project has multiple partners: the specialist palliative care team in the same acute hospital, the local hospice, a local primary care team, and the funding agency (the Irish Hospice Foundation). The aim of this chapter is to demonstrate how action research, and in particular the use of participatory action research (PAR), has enabled the development of palliative care interventions in acute respiratory care. It will also explore the importance of developing a communicative space with the multi-disciplinary team and will outline examples of action research cycles addressing this area.

The emphasis in PAR on collaboration, action, and reflection is particularly suited to this project given its multi-site, and multi-disciplinary nature. This project draws on Reason and Bradbury's definition of PAR as:

> A participatory, democratic process concerned with developing practical knowing in the pursuit of worthwhile human purposes, grounded in a participatory worldview . . . [and bringing] together action and reflection, theory and practice, in participation with others in the pursuit of practical solutions to issues of pressing concern and more generally the flourishing of individual persons and communities.
>
> (Reason and Bradbury, 2001: 1)

This study will demonstrate how PAR methods can support sharing and extending the practical knowing amongst healthcare professionals delivering palliative care.

Context

The establishment of the action research project was based on key recommendations in a report by the Health Service Executive and Irish Hospice Foundation (HSE/IHF, 2008): 'Palliative Care for All Implementing: Palliative Care into Disease Management Frameworks'. This report explored the provision of palliative care for people with diseases other than cancer from an Irish and international context. The report had a specific focus on advanced respiratory disease, heart failure, and dementia. Whilst there was overwhelming support in the literature for the need for palliative care, there was a dearth of service models to demonstrate how this could be achieved. To address this theory–practice gap, the Irish Hospice Foundation developed proposals for action research projects to be carried out with each disease speciality. The aim of these three projects was to devise, implement, and develop palliative care responses. Funding allowed for the employment of three part-time project officers over two years, introducing palliative interventions into clinical settings using an action research methodology. The research sites were selected through a competitive tendering process. Ethical approval was obtained from the relevant hospital and primary care bodies. This chapter recounts the experience of the advanced respiratory care project, which at the time of writing is still ongoing.

Developing the communicative space

Prior to the commencement of the advanced respiratory project, there were good relationships between the respiratory and palliative care teams, and an acceptance that patients with advanced respiratory disease warrant appropriate palliative care. These tentative beginnings were built upon through a collaborative approach that led to the successful tender for the project. Simultaneously, initial steps had been taken within the respiratory department's community outreach programme to extend it to include palliative care support. All of this meant that the early seeds of participation and a democratic process, to enable an action research approach, had been sown.

This early engagement enabled the formation of a communicative space (Kemmis, 2001) where dialogue could take place and relationships develop throughout the project timeframe. It is well recognized that this first step in action research (the formation of a communicative space) is central to action research and can influence the success of using this methodology (Gayá Wicks and Reason, 2009) (see Chapter 2). For this project the establishment of relationships with relevant stakeholders supported the rigour and scope of the work.

Within this project we sought to establish communicative spaces at a number of levels:

1. Regular steering committee meetings

   With the appointment of the project officer, a formal steering group consisting of eight key stakeholders was established. This group comprised of: a respiratory clinical nurse specialist, a consultant respiratory and general physician, a palliative care clinical nurse specialist, a palliative home care team manager, a consultant in palliative medicine, a general practitioner, the project officer, and the programme development manager from the Irish Hospice Foundation. These meetings take place approximately every eight weeks. After the first meeting, it was evident that this meeting time was unique and provided the opportunity for key personnel from the fields of respiratory and palliative care to form decisions and take actions.

2. Expert focus group

   Early on in the project, it became apparent that members of the steering group had not had the chance to openly discuss their understanding of the project and to reach a mutual understanding of how to progress it. With this in mind, the project

Box 9.1 Questions for the expert focus group.

1. What are your expectations for this project?
2. What outcomes would you like to see at the end of the two years?
3. Are there any potential barriers to achieving these?
   (a) What are they?
   (b) How can we overcome them?
4. What actions (action cycles) would you like to see happening?
5. What actions (action cycles) are realistic within the timeframe?
6. In what order/priority should they start?

officer suggested conducting the next steering group meeting as an expert focus group. This allowed for everyone to have the opportunity to engage meaningfully in the meeting and for consensus and collaboration to develop. The questions posed moved from broader questions on general expectations for the project to prioritizing action cycles (see Box 9.1).

This mechanism for developing the communicative space proved most worthwhile, as it allowed everyone to have a voice, and documented where they wanted the project to go. It was especially useful for the newly appointed research project officer to hear what everyone expected from the project. It was also evident from this early stage that there was openness to compromise and a willingness to work together as reported by these participants: 'Interested in how we work with respiratory team in using each other's specialist knowledge, improving communication or establishing good communication patterns there' (Specialist Palliative Care Nurse). 'Another thing is to disseminate the knowledge that we gain from working with each other in this close group to other staff involved in working with patients' (Respiratory Clinical Nurse Specialist). 'Hope that there would be a closer working relationship between the two different services, cross-fertilize a bit better . . . that's probably the difficult area' (Specialist Palliative Care Consultant).

3. Individual meetings

   An important mechanism for opening a communicative space was through the individual meetings the project officer held with key participants. Although this was time consuming, it was vital to the ongoing project as several team members were unable to maintain protected time for the project. It also allowed for other important stakeholders who were not in the steering committee to be included in the research, in particular the clinical nurse managers from the respiratory ward and the respiratory nurse specialists.

4. Visits to other sites

   The multi-site nature of the project meant that inclusion of the hospice and the primary care team required site visits. Even before the project had officially started there had been presentations and visits from the development staff of the Irish

Hospice Foundation and the respiratory nurse specialist to the home care teams in the hospice. A day of introductions had been planned for the project officer with key personnel in the hospice. These meetings provided valuable links with nursing and educational personnel. The project officer also met with the general practitioner at his practice several times and presented the project to the primary care team. Subsequent educational visits between hospice and acute hospital staff involved in the project have also been initiated.

5. Presentations to respiratory medical and nursing teams

It was also important that the respiratory teams (both medical and nursing) were informed and included in the project. Both the medical and nursing teams have weekly educational meetings and these were used to present the project at the beginning and to present results that emerged. These were valuable sessions to ensure that the participatory nature of action research was fostered, and as one nurse commented: 'This is the first time anyone's ever come back to tell us the results of something we filled out.'

Establishing palliative responses in respiratory care—using action cycles

One of the challenges that the action research posed was how to capture and hold all of the action cycles and dimensions of the project. Using a visual representation from early on in the project has helped to place all of the emerging components together in a meaningful way. The image of a tree was used as it has a solid trunk and roots—in the same way that the project had been well supported from the outset. Each of the actions—depicted as branches—whilst individual, all directly related back to the project (see Figure 9.1).

A number of action cycles were undertaken as part of this project (see Figure 9.1). Given the variety of developments that occurred within the project, two of the action cycles will be described here in more detail.

Education survey of palliative care needs

As previously mentioned, the pre-existing awareness from the ward staff of the need to change end-of-life care practices, has proved an efficacious catalyst for change. This realization of the need for change reflected the high clinical practice standards held on the ward, but required an enabler to put it into action. Here the value of the experiential knowing of the clinical staff complemented the propositional knowing (Reason, 2006) of the project officer. It allowed for time to reflect on the clinical experiences and developments. It was in this realm that the outsider role of the project officer was beneficial. Being an outsider of both the medical and nursing hierarchies, the project officer was perceived as non-threatening, respectful of workload, and enabled the pace of change to be led by the staff.

From early on in the process, arising from the expert focus group and meetings with the other project officers, it became apparent that education would be playing a key role in the project. In order to understand the educational needs of staff in the ward a

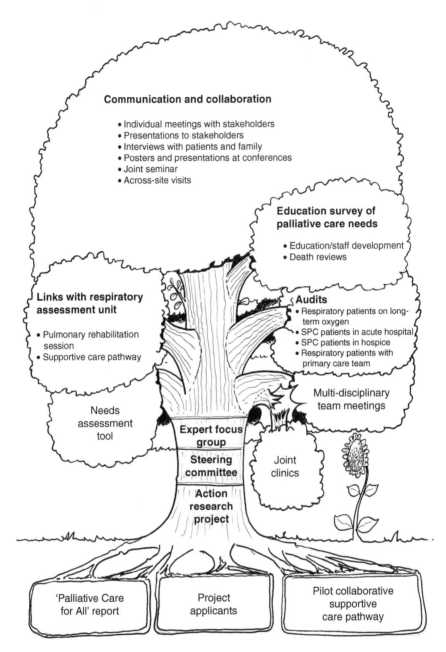

Fig. 9.1 Tree representation of project.
Image created by cassidycomics.com. Used with permission of Patricia White and Marie Lynch.

previously published questionnaire (McDonnell *et al.*, 2009) was used to clarify their specific requirements. The willingness of the clinical nurse managers to take on the data collection ensured an 86% response rate after two weeks. The analysis showed the participants held a view that palliative care was centred on care of the dying patient. Only 7% of staff had any further training or education in palliative care and 91% reported that they would be interested in attending a course on palliative care. The other major finding was that over half of the respondents felt there was no support after a patient dies and 82% felt this was an area that needed further development.

Within the education action cycle two specific actions were undertaken. The first action involved a programme of palliative care education specifically tailored for respiratory staff, which was developed through meetings with the palliative care nurse and personnel from the hospice foundation (see Table 9.1). The close links with the hospice foundation allowed for the use of training resources they had developed for another programme. At the time of writing, 22 respiratory staff members had completed the first two components of training and evaluations showed that it was very positively received by those who attended. However, no members of the respiratory medical teams had participated.

The second action arose from the education survey and feedback from the staff development programme. It has involved setting up a meeting time specifically for retrospective reviews of patients who have died. These have been called 'death review meetings' and have been developed from work by Hockley (Hockley and Froggatt, 2006). The aim is for staff to have the time to acknowledge the person who has died and reflect on their time with them, to examine what went well and to see if there is anything that could be changed to improve their care of dying patients. A constant theme from those working on the ward was that the busyness of a ward in an acute setting does not allow for time after someone dies, as stated by one nurse: 'It's onto the next task.' There have been two initial death review meetings attended by a

Table 9.1 Plan for education/staff development in palliative care

	Target audience	Duration	Facilitator	Progress
Developing awareness in end-of-life care	All respiratory staff	3 hours	Trained facilitator	Completed by 22 respiratory staff
Developing communication skills in end-of-life care	All respiratory staff	3 hours	Trained facilitator	Completed by 22 respiratory staff
Symptom management in advanced respiratory disease	Nursing and medical respiratory staff	1 hour	Member of specialist palliative care team	Date still to be confirmed
Breaking bad news	Nursing and medical respiratory staff	3 hours	Trained facilitator	Currently at pilot stage

total of 11 nurses. There has been a lack of engagement from the medical teams; however, it is hoped that this will be addressed. From discussions together, one approach could be to reframe the meetings as a more familiar medical death conference, where medical and psychosocial aspects are discussed for learning and continuous professional development purposes.

Using multi-disciplinary team meetings to assist collaboration

A second action cycle has been the development of a strong relationship between the respiratory teams and the specialist palliative care teams in the acute hospital and in the local hospice. At the start of the project there had been a patient with advanced respiratory disease who was successfully linked in with the hospice and their home care team. The nurses from both sites involved in this patient's care were important catalysts to relationship building and change. This has been facilitated by joint working on writing up the case history for a poster and presentation at national conferences and is currently being prepared for publication.

The development of shared care between the respiratory team and the hospice has been further progressed through the establishment of monthly multi-disciplinary, multi-site team meetings. Members of the respiratory and palliative care medical and nursing teams from the hospital attend, along with the advanced nurse practitioner from the hospice. This is a brief meeting of 30 minutes where, on average, five cases are presented. The most valuable aspect of these meetings is the update of information on patients to the various teams (see Figure 9.2). At times the medical staff have been unavailable to attend and this has limited the scope of the meetings. From early observations, there has been a shift in referral timing, with respiratory staff referring earlier in the disease pathway. A SCOT analysis (strengths, challenges, opportunities and threats) is currently underway with attendees to evaluate the meetings and a follow-up audit on all sites will be conducted to analyse changes in referral practices.

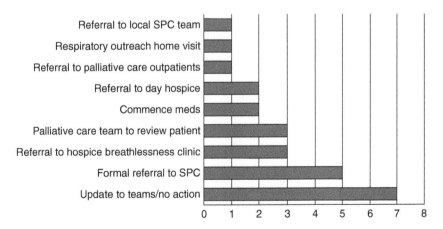

Fig. 9.2 Frequency of outcomes from first five multi-disciplinary meetings.

Challenges—enablers and inhibitors

There were many factors which enabled the development of a communicative space and subsequent action cycles. Alongside the steering committee and their commitment to the project, the clinical nurse managers on the respiratory ward and the respiratory clinical nurse specialists proved to be valuable contributors and collaborators. They fully engaged with the project, and the project officer met with them on a regular basis. The protected role of project officer in facilitating this shift within the context of the busy hierarchal clinical world has been central to this process. It was here that the benefits of an action research project embedded within an acute setting could be seen.

Naturally, due to the physical location of the project in the acute hospital setting there was a closer working relationship between the respiratory nurses and the palliative care nurses in the acute setting, than those based in the hospice. Often the casual meeting for lunch proved to be far more insightful and supportive than any number of formally arranged meetings. In particular, the relationship between the project officer and the respiratory clinical nurse specialist provided mutual support and multiple opportunities for the project to grow. The commitment of the respiratory nurse to the project was a fundamental factor in opening up space for communication and relationship building. She provided a consistent interface between the world of research and the clinically focused world of an acute hospital. The project officer and respiratory nurse endeavoured to have regular weekly meetings and these meetings have proved to be an important communicative space in its own right.

This project also benefited from the ongoing engagement with the Irish Hospice Foundation funder. Their support went far beyond a financial grant. They provided information support, access to literature, practical support, and, most importantly, they provided the space for monthly action learning sets where the three project officers could meet in a safe space to discuss critical and confidential issues (McGill and Brockbank, 2004). Given the isolating nature of action research, these meetings had an important role to play, particularly as relationships and trust built up over time.

As expected, there were also inhibitors to the development of a communicative space at all levels. The most dominant and persistent one was the available time people had and this was recognized early on as a barrier from the focus group held with steering group members: 'I think time is going to be a big barrier, even just to get here today' (clinician—senior nurse); 'I thought I wouldn't make it here today' (clinician—clinical nurse specialist); and, 'Finding space in the working week to make this a priority and resources to some extent' (clinician—medical). There was never a meeting time that was ideal for everyone and clinical demands meant that often at short notice, medical members of the team could not attend. Despite this, there was an average attendance of six people at each steering committee meeting. When members missed meetings, the project officer engaged with them on an individual level. The purpose of this was two-fold: first, to update them on the project, and second, to explore reasons for non-attendance which may lie beyond practical arrangements.

During the timeframe of the project, there were further financial cutbacks from the Health Service Executive which meant that staff who left, or were on leave of absence, were not replaced. This resulted in a noticeable increase in people's workload and priorities were given to more immediate clinical matters. In addition, one of the key stakeholders retired during the course of the project and, although they continued to support the project, this led to a leadership and expertise vacuum exacerbated by the delay in the appointment of their replacement.

An evident inhibitor when conducting action research in a medical setting is the conflicting research philosophies and health-illness perspectives that people have and how these impact on constructive relationships. These largely stem from differing professional epistemologies (Engel, 1977) and impacted upon the project in several ways. Firstly, there was a lack of understanding of action research. For some, this did not prove problematic to the running of the project. However, for others, accustomed to taking part in clinical trials with power calculated participant numbers and clearly measureable predefined outcomes, action research seemed intangible and elusive. The second epistemological difference was more noticeable on a wider scale rather than being present within the steering committee group. It relates to the disease management approach to advanced respiratory disease that dominates patient care, even at the end of life. It is a dichotomous approach which sees chronic disease management on the one hand and palliative care on the other, rather than incorporating palliative care throughout the patients' experience of their illness. This integrative concept of continuous palliation throughout chronic disease management (Gott *et al.*, 2009) is in its early stages.

What became apparent during the project was that there is the larger respiratory care culture in the hospital, consisting of several medical teams who still work from a disease management perspective. Alongside this is the world of the nurses on the ward who understand, embrace, and practice palliative care, but can, at times, be frustrated by the clinical decisions made by medical teams (Vejlgaard and Addington Hall, 2005). Finally, there is the sub-group of the respiratory assessment unit consisting of a consultant, physiotherapist, and nurses who provide community and supportive care to respiratory patients. This group, like the nurses, has taken on board and practice the principles of palliative care. They operate in a more independent manner because they are not located on the ward, making it easier to integrate care across settings (Hagg-Grün *et al.*, 2010).

These differing epistemologies exist within the power layers of medical hierarchy. This project took place within that hierarchy and so is not exempt from the cultural norms of power that exist within nursing and medical hierarchies. It was a frustration for the project officer that whilst the nurses were supportive and taking on changes within their nursing world, not all of the medical teams were fully embracing a palliative approach to care.

A further challenge has been the timeframe for the study. The ambitious timeframe of two years has now been extended by six months. It will not be long enough to constructively engage with all of the stakeholders, in particular, with primary care. This has been for practical resource reasons; however, there have been the beginnings of participatory relationships with members of the primary care team. It is these relationships that can now be built upon and used to examine how to facilitate the engagement of primary care in the future.

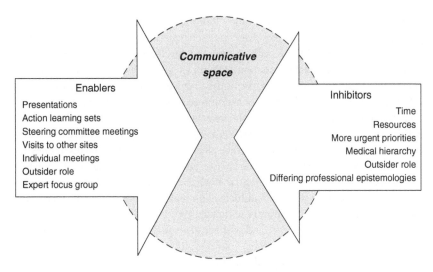

Fig. 9.3 Enablers and inhibitors of the communicative space.

The range of influences on the development of the communicative space in this project is visually demonstrated in Figure 9.3.

Discussion and reflections

Using the principles of action research allows for the examination of the research beyond its own outcomes to the wider social, cultural, and historical influencers. This has been helpful in understanding the impact of this project within the larger macro-cosm of respiratory and palliative care developments. As Reason (2006) discusses, there is a need to look beyond our own piece of work to creating social movements. Indeed, this project, whilst on a small scale, is part of a greater national and international move to broaden palliative care into the care of people with non-malignant diseases. At a local level, knowledge of this new approach has been disseminated through meetings and presentations to teams within the hospital and hospice. At a national and international level, the project is being presented at respiratory and palliative care conferences. This contributes to the dialogue on extending palliative care for all life-limiting illnesses. There are also synergies with the work that has been conducted by Geralyn Hynes (see Chapter 15), and it is encouraging that action research is playing its role in the momentum of change in palliative care for advanced respiratory patients.

Action research also requires an historical perspective and this has been helpful when faced with the challenge of changing medical practice. Understanding that palliative care is a relatively new speciality and is even still being accepted and integrated into oncology (Cherny and Catane, 2003) has helped maintain a perspective on the expectations of this project. Furthermore, bringing about change in any organization takes time (Henderson and McKillop, 2008) and it has been recognized within practice development that it takes five years to change culture. Taking this longitudinal perspective is in line with the evolutionary and developmental process that is at the heart of the emergent quality of action research (Reason, 2006). It would therefore be helpful to revisit the project site in the future to evaluate the legacy of this work.

Critical reflection is at the heart of action research and supports overall consideration of overall learning process from the project (Reil, 2010). The use of action research in this project has helped the author (PW) as the project officer to achieve two things. First, it allowed for communication to take place amongst and between disciplines and sites. This process has led to a transformative process of reflection and action, which highlights Friere's (1975) epistemology, that when action and reflection occur simultaneously they become creative and mutually illuminate each other. It can be seen in this quote from the project: 'Respiratory and palliative care knowledge based values and world views have come together and we have generated a new practice based knowledge base' (Clinical Nurse Specialist). Second, it has enabled the author to see the project from a phenomenological standpoint. The project does not exist in isolation, rather within a complex local, political, economic, and cultural context. This has been hugely helpful in dealing with the setbacks and frustrations that characterize research.

Reflection methods used by the funder representative (ML) included personal note taking following meetings and key milestones, as well as participation in the action learning set. The reflective process was critical in helping the author (as funder) maintain reasonable expectations for the project, and be perceptive and subsequently supportive to the project through some of its challenging transitions.

Conclusion

At the core of this project is bridging the theory practice gap between the palliative care approach and the management of advanced respiratory disease. This meant that the task-oriented, urgent nature of daily clinical practice met with the often ethereal world of action research. Despite the collisions that ensued along the way, the integration of theory and practice did occur within the communicative space that had developed. Central to this was the existing desire to improve practice so that the palliative needs of patients with advanced respiratory disease could be acknowledged and responded to within the parameters of the respiratory service, ultimately providing a more holistic approach to care.

References

Cherny, N.I. and Catane, R. (2003) Attitudes of Medical Oncologists toward Palliative Care for Patients with Advanced and Incurable Cancer. *Cancer*, **98**: 2502–10.

Engel, G.L. (1977) The Need for a New Medical Model: A Challenge for Biomedicine. *Science*, **196**: 129–36.

Freire, P. (1975) *Education: The Practice of Freedom*, p. 147. London: Writers and Readers Publishing Co-operative.

Gayá Wicks, P. and Reason, P. (2009) Initiating Action Research: Challenges and Paradoxes of Opening Communicative Space. *Action Research*, **7**(3): 243–62.

Gott, M., Gardiner, C., Small, N., et al. (2009) Barriers to Advance Care Planning in Chronic Obstructive Pulmonary Disease. *Palliative Medicine*, **23**(7): 642–48.

Hagg-Grün, U., Lukas, A., Sommer, B.N., Klaiber, H.R., and Nikolaus T. (2010) Implementation of a Palliative Care Concept in a Geriatric Acute Care Hospital. *Zeitschrift für Gerontologie und Geriatrie*, **43**(6): 362–8.

Henderson, L. and McKillop, S. (2008) Using Practice Development Approaches in the Development of a Managed Clinical Network. In: K. Manley, B. McCormack, and V. Wilson (eds), *International Practice Development in Nursing and Healthcare*, pp. 319–48. Oxford: Blackwell Publishing.

Hockley, J. (2006) *Developing High Quality End of Life Care in Nursing Care Homes: An Action Research Study.* Unpublished PhD thesis, University of Edinburgh.

Hockley, J. and Froggatt, K. (2006) The Development of Palliative Care Knowledge in Care Homes for Older People: The Place of Action Research. *Palliative Medicine*, **20**: 835–43.

Irish Hospice Foundation and Health Service Executive (IHF/HSE) (2008) *Palliative Care for All Implementing: Palliative Care into Disease Management Frameworks.* Dublin: Irish Hospice Foundation and Health Service Executive.

Kemmis, S. (2001) Exploring the Relevance of Critical Theory for Action Research: Emancipatory Action Research in The Footsteps Of Jürgen Habermas. In: P. Reason and H. Bradbury (eds), *Handbook of Action Research: Participative Inquiry and Practice*, pp. 91–102. London: Sage.

McDonnell, M.M., McGuigan, E., McElhinney, J., McTeggart, M., and McClure, D. (2009) An Analysis of the Palliative Care Education Needs of RGNs and HCAs in Nursing Homes in Ireland. *International Journal of Palliative Nursing*, **15**(9): 446, 448–55.

McGill, I. and Brockbank, A. (2004) *Action Learning Handbook*: Powerful Techniques for Education, Training and Professional Development. London: Routledge Farmer.

Reason, P. (2006) Choice and Quality in Action Research Practice. *Journal of Management Inquiry*, **15**(2): 187–203.

Reason, P. and Bradbury-Huang, H. (2001) Inquiry and Participation in Search of a World Worthy of Human Aspiration. In: P. Reason and H. Bradbury (eds), *Handbook of Action Research: Participative Inquiry and Practice*, pp. 1–14. London: Sage.

Riel, M. (2010) *Understanding Action Research.* Centre For Collaborative Action Research. Pepperdine University. Available at: http://cadres.pepperdine.edu/ccar/define.html (accessed 16 January 2012).

Vejlgaard, T. and Addington-Hall, J.M. (2005) Attitudes of Danish Doctors and Nurses to Palliative and Terminal Care. *Palliative Medicine*, **19**(2): 119–27.

Chapter 10

Improving pain management in Canadian long-term care homes

Sharon Kaasalainen

As the population continues to age, more people will die in long-term care (LTC), with estimates as high as 39% of residents dying in their LTC home annually by the year 2020 (Fisher *et al.*, 2000). Unlike other sectors, most LTC residents die from non-cancer conditions, with one study reporting that only 14% of deaths were due to cancer (Hall *et al.*, 2002). Within LTC, up to 75% of residents have cognitive impairment (Proctor and Hirdes, 2001), which creates additional challenges to providing effective palliative care due to the related cognitive, communication, functional, and behavioural problems that arise (Kaasalainen *et al.*, 2007a; Sachs *et al.*, 2004).

One of the most common symptoms at the end of life is pain, which can cause the greatest suffering for individuals (Hall *et al.*, 2002). Pain management for older adults in LTC, particularly those with cognitive impairment, has been recognized as an international problem (Zwakhalen *et al.*, 2009). Rates of pain in LTC homes are as high as 83% and it has been identified in some LTC settings that approximately 4% of residents experience daily pain that is excruciating (Boerlage *et al.*, 2008; Teno *et al.*, 2004; Zwakhalen *et al.*, 2009). Despite the high rates, pain continues to be under-assessed and under-treated in the older adult population living in LTC homes (Mitchell *et al.*, 2003; Won *et al.*, 2004). Efforts are needed to improve pain management within this vulnerable population.

In this chapter, a description of an action-based model to improve pain management in long-term care (Kaasalainen *et al.*, 2010) will be discussed, along with its development and validation. Interventions or actions that were guided by this model will be presented and an evaluation of them highlighted.

Development of the model

This model was developed within the context of a larger project that evolved from a mutual interest in improving pain management in LTC. Specifically, I, the researcher wanted to implement an intervention to improve the way pain was managed, and two partnering LTC homes were driven by a need to improve pain care processes to meet provincial regulatory requirements. Through our collaborative efforts, funding was received to implement and evaluate a pain protocol at the two LTC homes, so our partnership became more formalized as we sought to produce, 'knowledge and action directly useful to a community' (Reason, 1994: 48). Knowing that the process of implementing the pain protocol would be demanding for staff amidst many barriers within a challenging social system, the decision was made to use a participatory action research approach to build capacity and empower staff throughout the project (Kidd and Kral, 2005). Guided by a critical theory framework, a social or situational analysis was undertaken alongside the self-study of current practices in pain management, and how language was used, while keeping in mind the organization and power within these two LTC homes (Kemmis and McTaggart, 2000). The end goal was to develop actions to produce change and improve the way pain was currently being managed, with a constructive and positive manner (Kemmis and McTaggart, 2000; Reason, 1994).

The situational analysis included a number of interviews, focus groups, and a short survey about the barriers to managing pain in LTC, which was completed by health-care providers and managers who worked at the two LTC homes. Using a semi-structured interview guide, interview questions focused on eliciting information about current practices relating to pain management and some of the barriers and facilitators to providing effective pain management for residents. The intent was to gather information that was rich and free-flowing; we therefore purposely interviewed different types of care providers and members of the administrative team separately, so we could tap into their perspectives about their relationships and interactions with other care providers and other LTC staff. Once all of the interviews were conducted, transcribed and analysed using thematic content analysis, we developed an initial draft of the model in response to the data that emerged. The model underwent much iteration based on feedback from a variety of individuals, as discussed in more detail below.

Methods undertaken to validate the model

A number of approaches to validate the model and ensure rigour in the methodology were used. These approaches were reflexive in nature and 'formed over time through dialectic movement between action and reflection' (Kidd and Kral, 2005: 187). To do this, forums were organized with various groups of individuals where dialogue was initiated about the components of the model, as well as their experiences related to it, so that the actions listed in the model were collectively endorsed (Kidd and Kral, 2005).

First, the initial analysis was summarized in a two-page format that was shared with all participants, including residents and family members, with a request for feedback. The draft model was presented at a resident council and a family council meeting to elicit further feedback. No recommendations for changes were put forward at this time but rather their responses confirmed that the strategies listed were important ones.

The draft of the model was also shared and presented with each LTC home separately at meetings with all levels of staff. Based on feedback that was received from them, certain elements of the model were modified. For example, the original draft combined the residents and family members together but staff felt that these two groups had unique challenges with regards to pain management, and therefore strategies undertaken to improve pain management would differ as well. Hence the next version of the model kept residents at the core, with family members at the next level outward. Second, staff confirmed the importance of keeping unregulated care providers (UCPs), otherwise called personal support workers (PSWs), separated from the regulated care providers and being positioned closest to families and residents, since PSWs spend most of the time at the bedside and they reiterated the importance of the PSW role in managing pain. Also, staff recognized the importance of the subsequent levels (licensed healthcare providers, organization, system) to empower and build capacity within PSWs. The PSWs also felt that they should be separated out from the licensed health-care providers since they have more direct contact with family members and residents and generally see themselves as a team on their own. Staff at one of the homes high-lighted the need to incorporate education about pain management in the orientation of new staff (this item was not included in the initial draft) due to high staff turnover. Hence, this was included in subsequent versions of the model. The need for inclusion of this item was later confirmed by the other LTC home as well.

Following revisions to the model based on the feedback, the literature was searched to confirm that the strategies recommended in the model were inclusive and consist-ent with other studies and best practice guidelines. In addition, the model was pre-sented at a forum hosted by the Ontario Ministry of Health and Long Term Care that included over 50 governmental employers who were largely responsible for overseeing the regulation of LTC homes in Ontario. At this time, the suggestion to include gov-ernmental regulations that specifically addressed pain management in the model was recommended (this item was not included in earlier drafts of the model). Hence, this item was added to the model under the 'system' category.

Description of the model

The action-based model to improve pain management in LTC includes six levels, with corresponding interventions proposed at each level: resident, family, unregulated care providers, licensed care providers, organization, and system (see Figure 10.1). Within this model, residents comprise the focal point with all other layers influencing how resident pain is managed, but those that are closest to the resident having the most direct interaction. At the resident level, attention needs to be focused on encouraging residents to report their pain consistently to healthcare providers so that their pain can be managed effectively.

The model highlights that every effort should be focused on encouraging residents to disclose their pain and at the very least to report the presence of it to staff. Pain can mean different things to different people. Given this, care should be focused on individualiz-ing both the assessment of pain and its treatment. It is important to allow residents a choice of assessment tool to report their pain as preferences vary. Once a resident has chosen a particular scale, then that scale should be used consistently in their care. In this manner, pain reporting can become normalized in care routines and any fluctuations of pain can be tracked well over time, ideally when there is a change in status or before and after a pain treatment has been administered. Once pain has been detected, then resi-dents should be involved in decisions related to how it will be treated or managed.

When residents are not able to verbally report their pain, as in the case of people with severe dementia or stroke, family members need to act as a proxy for pain report-ing. Family members generally have an intimate knowledge of their relatives in terms

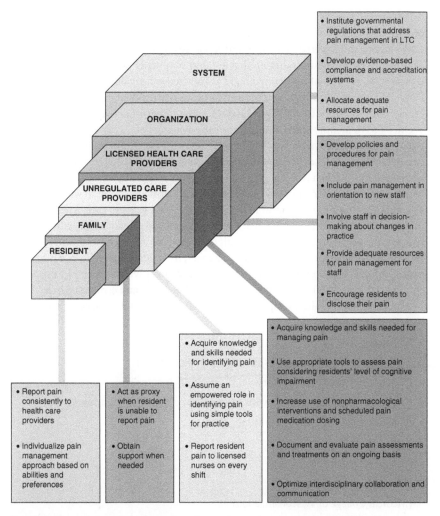

Fig. 10.1 An action-based approach to improving pain management in long-term care.
Reproduced with permission from Kaasalainen, S. *et al.*, An action-based approach to improving
pain management in long-term care. *Canadian Journal on Aging*, **29**(4): 503–17
© Cambridge University Press 2010.

of their normal habits, pain tolerance, chronic conditions, and can provide rich history about their relative, along with preferences for care. Family members should be involved in setting goals for residents if needed. Like residents, family members also need information to help them feel empowered and involved in decision making. It is important to gain a sense of what the goals are for family members compared to residents and if their goals differ. Types of goals that are important to family members might include residents' comfort level, desired balance of comfort, and other side effects of pain medications, such as alertness.

Personal support workers (PSWs) comprise the largest group of staff in LTC and provide the majority of bedside care, yet have the least amount of training. Unfortunately, PSWs are not empowered to identify and report resident pain to supervising nurses in an effective manner. Efforts are needed to build supportive supervisory relationships so that PSW reports of resident pain are acknowledged. By building capacity within PSWs to improve the way they identify and report resident pain, better working relationships between the PSWs and their nursing supervisors may result.

Once PSWs identify when a resident is experiencing pain, licensed healthcare providers (i.e. nurses, physicians, allied health team members) play an important role in conducting further assessments and implementing and evaluating treatments aimed at alleviating pain. When residents are no longer able to make decisions for themselves, which is commonplace in LTC, licensed health care providers need to work with family members to a larger extent to make decisions about goals of care. These kinds of decisions are difficult to make, particularly those related to pain management. Often typical pain behaviours are confused with other conditions, such as delirium, depression, or a result of dementia itself. In these cases, treatment often follows a pragmatic approach, which generally begins with a course of anti-psychotics, and by process of elimination, pain medications may be prescribed in a trial and error approach.

Education about pain management across all levels of staff is needed and should include information about:

- Types of pain
- Common beliefs and attitudes about pain in older adults
- Conducting a basic pain history
- Pain assessment for residents with and without cognitive impairment
- Non-pharmacological interventions
- Basic analgesic pharmacology
- Analgesic algorithms
- Communicating the message

    (Medical College of Wisconsin, 2000)

At the organization level, LTC homes need to make pain management a priority. In doing so, policies and procedures related to pain management are needed and education should be provided for all new staff at orientation training and for continuing education using 'top-up' sessions for all levels of staff. Interventions are needed to facilitate a supportive environment for residents to feel comfortable disclosing and discussing their pain with LTC staff. At the same time, healthcare providers need to engage and advocate for residents to report their pain. If the organization presents a 'pain-friendly' environment, perhaps residents will be more comfortable talking about their pain.

At the system level, there is a need to develop and institute governmental regulations that specifically address pain management in LTC, which then provide the basis for the development and implementation of evidence-based compliance and accreditation systems. In order for LTC homes to be able to meet these standards, adequate resources for pain management need to be allocated to them.

Actions driven by the model

This model continues to be used to develop innovative strategies to improve the way pain is managed in LTC, while taking into account the pervasive barriers and facilitators that exist in this sector. Consistent with a participatory action research approach, these strategies/actions involved a series of cycles of reflection, planning, acting, and observing (McTaggart, 1997). For example, an interdisciplinary pain protocol intervention was developed based on recommendations of the model, which included an educational workshop to launch the intervention, the use of simple pain assessment tools, an interdisciplinary pain flow sheet to promote better communication about resident pain across all levels of staff, and development/refinement of institutional policies and procedures specific to pain management. Evaluation results of this intervention revealed that pain increased significantly more ($F = 5.92$; $p = 0.016$) for residents in the control group, compared to the intervention group (Kaasalainen *et al.*, 2012). When asked to provide recommendations to improve the protocol, most participants stated that it involved too much paperwork and that it needed to be simplified, and its documentation be reduced. It was also suggested that the admission/initial pain assessment form be used quarterly, or when there is a change in a resident's health status.

Another project focused on building capacity within the PSW role to identify pain using simple tools and then reporting it to licensed nurses in a timely manner. It involved providing education about pain in LTC and ways to manage it better, and skills training about how to use simple pain assessment tools correctly. Evaluation of this intervention is forthcoming but anecdotal comments from both PSWs and managers indicate that the intervention was successful in engaging and empowering PSWs to identify resident pain and communicate it effectively to licensed nurses.

In Ontario, Canada, in 2010, a new pain management programme was included as one of six programmes mandated within the new Ontario Regulations Under the 2007 Long Term Care Act (Ontario Ministry of Health and Long Term Care, 2010). As a result, LTC homes across the province are required to meet these new pain standards in order to pass the inspection process. It is hoped that instituting the new pain management programme will serve as a catalyst to improve pain management practices in LTC homes in Ontario. By endorsing a commitment to improving pain management at the system level, it encourages change at all other levels of care as well, as depicted in the action based model to improve pain management in long-term care.

Currently, work is also being done in partnership with a provincial organization that provides support to LTC homes to improve quality care by providing access to resources and supporting LTC homes to implement practice changes. The goal of our partnership is to develop a toolkit based on the action-based model to improve pain management in LTC. As such, an advisory board comprised of 26 experts in the field that are representative of all interdisciplinary groups from the LTC sector (i.e. LTC administrators, physicians, pharmacists, licensed nurses, PSWs, healthcare educators, representatives from Concerned Friends, and the Residents Councils of Ontario), has met three times to prioritize key 'change ideas' based on the pain model. With this group, we utilized a Delphi survey technique to identify and prioritize key change ideas guided by the pain model, with each change idea rated for both feasibility and importance. We chose to use a Delphi technique to ensure that the voices of all members of the advisory board are heard and to reach consensus within this very diverse group of individuals. Results of from the Delphi survey depicting key change ideas are pending.

Next steps

It is our intent to build a toolkit for LTC homes that can be easily accessed through a common portal hosted by the partnering organization who will also help to disseminate it. This toolkit is intended for a number of target audiences, namely LTC organizations, administrators, healthcare providers, and other decision-makers. We will work closely with policy makers to ensure that the toolkit addresses the new regulations and compliance standards appropriately, but this initiative is seen as most useful to those working in the LTC sector. This work will help disseminate and provide easy access to these recommended tools to avoid each home struggling to find these tools on their own or even worse, implementing pain assessment tools that are not evidence based.

We anticipate challenges with continued implementation of the action based model to improve pain management in long-term care, including a number of barriers to the uptake of the pain toolkit, such as heavy nursing workload, competing demands, personal values and beliefs about pain, initial resistance to change, reluctance or lack of confidence to try something new, lack of resources, and challenges assessing and managing pain in LTC (Kaasalainen *et al.*, 2007b; Martin *et al.*, 2005). For example, despite the pain toolkit, clinician beliefs and attitudes about pain may influence their decision making regarding pain management and treatment options within LTC settings. Research has indicated that opioid medications are under utilized in seniors, particularly those with cognitive impairment (Morrison and Siu, 2000). Weissman and Matson (1999) found a widespread fear of treating pain without understanding the exact cause of pain, along with concern about over-medication and drug toxicity, especially for those seniors with cognitive impairment.

Bowers *et al.* (2001) found that nurses' workload and attitude towards work were impacted by time and suggested that time constraints limit nurses in their ability to implement changes to their practice, such as improving pain management practices. Moreover, Resnick *et al.* (2004) found that workload demands related to documentation were a common challenge when implementing clinical practice guidelines (CPGs) within 23 LTC facilities and as a result, recommended keeping it short and sweet.

However, the toolkit will include resources and recommendation to overcome some of the barriers. Moreover, the urgency to update and revise their current pain management policies and procedures to meet the new compliance standards will create a strong impetus, particularly for LTC administrators, to access and use the toolkit to meet these standards. Therefore the timing of this action-based initiative could not be better, which will increase the probability of the uptake of the toolkit within the LTC sector.

Conclusion

In summary, pain management is an important component in providing quality palliative care to LTC residents. However, many barriers exist that preclude optimal pain management in this unique setting. By using a PAR approach, the action based model to improve pain management in long-term care offers suggestions to focus on in order to address barriers at multiple levels within the healthcare system. It is hope that addressing these barriers within a mutli-faceted approach will lead to capacity development within the LTC sector and improved resident outcomes, particularly relating to pain management, may be realized.

References

Boerlage, A., van Dijk, M., Stronks, D., de Wit, R., and van der Rijt, C. (2008) Pain Prevalence and Characteristics in Three Dutch Residential Homes. *European Journal of Pain*, **12**: 910–16.

Bowers, B.J., Lauring, C., and Jacobson, N. (2001) How Nurses Manage Time and Work in Long Term Care. *Journal of Advanced Nursing*, **33**(4): 484–91.

Fisher, F., Ross, M., and MacLean, M. (2000) *A Guide to End-of-Life Care for Seniors*. Toronto, Canada: University of Toronto and University of Ottawa.

Hall, P., Schroder, C., and Weaver, L. (2002) The Last 48 Hours of Life in Long Term Care: A Focused Chart Audit. *Journal of the American Geriatrics Society*, **50**: 501–6.

Kaasalainen, S., Brazil, K., Coker, E., et al. (2010) An Action-Based Approach to Improving Pain Management in Long Term Care. *Canadian Journal on Aging*, **29**(4): 503–17.

Kaasalainen, S., Brazil, K., Coker, E., et al. (2012) Implementation and Evaluation of an Interdisciplinary Pain Protocol in Long Term Care. *American Medical Directors Association* (in press).

Kaasalainen, S., Brazil, K., Ploeg, J., and Schindel, M.L. (2007a) Nursing Processes of Providing Palliative Care or Long Term Care Residents with Dementia. *Journal of Palliative Care*, **23**(3): 173–80.

Kaasalainen, S., Coker, E., Dolovich, L., et al. (2007b) Pain Management Decision-Making among Long-Term Care Physicians and Nurses. *Western Journal of Nursing Research*, **29**(5): 561–80.

Kemmis, S. and McTaggart, R. (2005) Participatory Action Research. In: N.K. Denzin and Y.S. Lincoln (eds), *Handbook of Qualitative Research*, pp. 559–603. Thousand Oaks, CA: Sage.

Kidd, S. and Kral, M. (2005) Practicing Participatory Action Research. *Journal of Counseling Psychology*, **52**(2): 187–95.

Martin, R., Williams, J., Hadjistavropoulos, T., Hadjistavropoulos, H., and MacClean, M. (2005) A Qualitative Investigation on Seniors' and Caregivers' Views on Pain Assessment and Management. *Canadian Journal of Nursing Research*, **37**(2): 142–64.

McTaggart, R. (1997) Guiding Principles for Participatory Action Research. In: R. McTaggart (ed.), *Participatory Action Research: International Contexts and Consequences*, pp. 25–44. New York: State University of New York.

Medical College of Wisconsin (2000) *Nursing Staff Education Resource Manual: Pain Management 101 for Long Term Care Facilities*. Milwaukee, WI: The Medical College of Wisconsin.

Mitchell, S., Teno, J., Roy, J. Kabumoto, G., and Mor, V. (2003) Clinical and Organizational Factors Associated with Feeding Tube Use among Nursing Home Residents with Advanced Cognitive Impairment. *JAMA*, **290**: 73–80.

Morrison, R. and Siu, A. (2000) A Comparison of Pain and its Treatment in Advanced Dementia and Cognitively Intact Patients with Hip Fractures. *Journal of Pain and Symptom Management*, **19**(4): 240–8.

Ontario Ministry of Health and Long Term Care (2010) *Ontario Regulation Under the Long Term Care Homes Act (2007)* available at: http://www.e-laws.gov.on.ca/html/source/regs/english/2010/elaws_src_regs_r10079_e.htm (accessed 28 October 2011).

Proctor, W. and Hirdes, J. (2001) Pain and Cognitive Status among Nursing Home Residents in Canada. *Pain Research Management*, **6**: 119–25.

Reason, P. (1994) Human Inquiry as Discipline and Practice. In: P. Reason (ed.), *Participation in Human Inquiry*, pp. 40–56. Thousand Oaks, CA: Sage.

Resnick, B., Quinn, C., and Baxter, S. (2004) Testing the Feasibility of Implementation of Clinical Practice Guidelines in LTC Facilities. *Journal of the American Medical Directors Association*, **5**(1): 1–8.

Sachs, G.A., Shega, J.W., and Cox-Hayley, D. (2004) Barriers to Excellent End of Life Care for Patients with Dementia. *Journal of General Internal Medicine*, **19**: 1057–63.

Teno, J., Kabumoto, G., Wetle, T., Roy, J., and Mor, V. (2004) Daily Pain that was Excruciating at Some Time in the Previous Week: Prevalence, Characteristics, and Outcomes in Nursing Home Residents. *Journal of the American Geriatrics Society*, **52**: 762–67.

Weissman, D. and Matson, S. (1999) Pain Assessment and Management in the Long Term Care Setting. *Theoretical Medicine*, **20**: 31–43.

Won, A., Lapane, K., Vallow, S., Schein, J., Morris, J., and Lipsitz, L. (2004) Persistent Non-Malignant Pain and Analgesic Prescribing Patterns in Elderly Nursing Home Residents. *Journal of the American Geriatrics Society*, **52**: 867–74.

Zwakhalen, S., Koopmans, R., Geels, P., Berger M.P.F., and Hamers, J.P.H. (2009) The Prevalence of Pain in Nursing Home Residents with Dementia Measured Using an Observational Pain Scale. *European Journal of Pain*, **13**(1): 89–93.

Section 3

Issues

Chapter 11

Power relations: enhancing the delivery of a palliative approach in an aged care setting

Sharon Andrews, Fran McInerney, and
Andrew Robinson

Introduction and background

In this chapter we report on a critical action research study that focused on the development of relationships between staff working in an aged care facility (ACF) in Australia and family members of people with dementia, in the context of a palliative approach to care. We highlight the complex operation of power relations within the aged care setting and how this impacts on the establishment of collaborative-reciprocal relationships between family members and staff, as well as the way in which power is implicit within the action research process.

This study was positioned against a background of demographic shifts in the Australian population (Australian Bureau of Statistics, 2008), which, like elsewhere in the world have contributed to people entering ACFs older, more dependent, and more likely to have some form of dementia (Andrews *et al.*, 2009; Knapp *et al.*, 2007). In conjunction with this, an emerging recognition that dementia is a terminal condition (Mitchell *et al.*, 2009) has resulted in a palliative approach to care being advocated as the best practice for people with dementia residing in ACFs (Australian Department of Health and Ageing, 2006). However, barriers such as family members' inadequate knowledge of dementia (Forbes *et al.*, 2000), inequitable relations between staff and family, and tensions about who has control over care processes (Haesler *et al.*, 2010) challenge the development of collaborative care partnerships.

Within ACFs more generally, contextual factors such as staffing arrangements, professional isolation (Andrews *et al.*, 2012), as well as regulatory and economic rationalist agendas (Angus and Nay, 2003), frustrate the adoption of best practice. For example, aged care staff work in a historically hierarchical staffing structure, where personal care staff experience the least autonomy, have minimal impact on decision making and are subordinate within a clearly defined nursing hierarchy (Jervis, 2002; Andrews *et al.*, 2012). These existing power relations produce rigid role demarcation (Andrews *et al.*, 2012), which can undermine possibilities for collaboration by regulating what can be said and by whom. Such issues impact on the capacity of aged care staff to engage with a best practice palliative approach to care. To address these problems it is imperative to understand the effects of power and how it is exercised through various discourses, practices, and institutional arrangements. This chapter reports on a study investigating ways that staff working in an ACF might develop practices around a palliative approach to care for people with dementia and their families using a critical action research methodology.

Theoretical perspectives

Action research approaches have been increasingly advocated as a means of facilitating practice development and generating knowledge in areas of palliative care and aged care (Froggatt *et al.*, 2006; Hockley, 2002). Underpinned by the tenets of critical social theory (see Chapter 2), critical action research specifically focuses on facilitating change in people's practices, their understandings of these, and conditions of practice (Kemmis, 2001: 95).This type of research has an overtly collaborative and critically reflective intent; and seeks to challenge dominant power relations with the goal of cultivating more equitable and just circumstances (Kincheloe and McLaren, 2008). The action research process operates through a recurring spiral involving planning, taking action, and collecting data, analysis, reflection, re-planning, and so on. Through this process, participants such as aged care staff can develop a sense of ownership of and responsibility for the problems they seek to address, as well as the research process itself (Street and Robinson, 1995).

Through collaborative and dialogic encounters, critical action research opens up possibilities for practitioners to engage in an analysis of the mechanisms of power in which taken for granted understandings and practices are invested (Robinson 1995: 68). Power can be understood not as 'held' but 'exercised' and it 'only exists in action' (Foucault, 1977: 89). From this perspective no person is exempt from the effects of power as it is exercised through day-to-day practices (Gaventa and Cornwall, 2001). Foucault (1977) argues that power has not only a repressive function but also productive features and is inextricably linked to knowledge such that it: 'Perpetually creates knowledge, and conversely, knowledge constantly induces the effects of power' (Foucault 1977: 52). It is through this knowledge/power nexus that certain truths are produced that support dominant interests (which in ACFs are often structured around efficiency) and give orientation to people's actions, which, in turn, sustain such interests.

A key focus of critical action research is to support people, such as aged care staff, to develop more critical understandings of the taken-for-granted conditions that define their practice in particular ways. Through participation in ongoing cycles of action, critical reflection, and critique, people can come to a new recognition of their complicity in sustaining unjust circumstances, and realize that they have the capacity to exercise power to challenge the status quo towards more just and equitable ends (Gaventa and Cornwell, 2001). It is this process of empowerment that is the ultimate aspiration of critical action research.

Challenges to establishing a collaborative agenda in aged care settings—issues of power

The collaborative imperative of action research is realized by mobilizing a diversity of viewpoints (Koch and Kralik, 2006) so that participants become active agents in the construction of knowledge about their world (Heron and Reason, 2001). However, asymmetrical power relations between the researcher and participants are often highlighted as a tension in conducting action research, which can frustrate the establishment of collaborative relationships (Mason and Boutilier, 1996). The researcher's elevated status as an expert (i.e. having command of research knowledge and skills) has the potential to disempower research participants. Indeed, within ACFs where staff may have limited exposure to collaborative forms of research (Andrews *et al.*, 2012), such relations can result in participants becoming dependent on the researcher to facilitate their engagement in the research process, or struggling to shift a researcher-set agenda. Power relations between the participants themselves can also be a barrier to the development of egalitarian relationships in the research process. To set up conditions that will support collaboration, participants who are research naive require some leadership and guidance from a facilitator/researcher to negotiate power relations and build their capacity to engage in the action research process (Andrews *et al.*, 2012). Strategies to address these issues are discussed below with reference to our project findings.

The project

Our project addressed the question: what are the possibilities for developing the practice of aged care staff around a palliative approach to care for people with dementia and their family members? It was conducted in one dementia secure unit (DSU) that accommodated between 35 and 40 people with advanced dementia within a larger ACF. In keeping with the collaborative imperative of critical action research, an action research group (ARG) was established. Five members of approximately 35 staff on the unit volunteered to be part of the ARG: two Registered Nurses (RNs), one Enrolled Nurse (EN) and two personal care assistants (PCAs). Regular ARG meetings provided a primary source of data, used later in this chapter. Meetings were recorded and transcribed. The transcripts were developed into meeting notes to provide a first level analysis of the group's discussions. The notes were returned to the group prior to each successive meeting, in order to facilitate their critical reflection on emerging issues. During the three stages of the project the ARG moved through a number of action cycles which focused on exploring members' current practices, understanding the experiences of family members, and addressing the information and support needs of families.

Stage 1: Preliminary investigation—a facilitated engagement

Entering the field

In this project the researchers entered the field with a predefined question, and the impetus for the study was clearly researcher-driven at the early stages. Given that the ARG members had never before been part of an action research project, it was important to address issues of power implicit in the relationship between the researcher and the group members, and build their capacity to engage in the research process. Therefore, in one of the early ARG meetings the first author (SA) provided an introductory education session about action research processes and the project goals. The intention of this session was to familiarize the group members with the action research approach and to engage the group to think about their position in the research. This activity began an early conversation between participants about how they might work with SA and each other to investigate their practice. Additionally, in acknowledgement of the existing hierarchal relationships between staff on the DSU, group members were also encouraged by SA to develop a set of rules to guide discussions so that each member had an equal opportunity and felt able to speak freely during their meetings. This supported group members to openly discuss what they considered to be important issues influencing the delivery of a palliative approach to care. While SA was present to clarify concerns and, at times, ask probing questions to encourage the group members to critically reflect on certain issues, the group determined the course of the discussion. Hence, the group members' dialogic encounters shaped the issues to be addressed and therefore the direction of the project from an early stage.

Issues impacting on practice

During the early meetings, the ARG identified a range of issues constraining the delivery of a palliative approach to care on the DSU. Heavy work demands and documentation requirements were identified as key factors driving the construction of instrumental and routine care on the unit. Catherine, one of the PCAs in the group, explained that in order to meet heavy work demands her practice was necessarily task-orientated. She described it as 'repetitive' and 'remote control'. Similarly, Elizabeth (another personal care assistant (PCA)) argued, 'There is no time for one on one [resident] care.' Anne (EN) added that the competing demands of heavy workloads and time constraints meant that the emotional needs of family members were often neglected: 'We've got a new resident and … her daughter is really grieving at the moment. I spent about half an hour on Monday night with her on the phone … and … I'm trying to get off the phone, knowing that I had to be down on [another unit] … you just don't have the time' (EN). Despite such realizations the group members' discussions revealed that staff-family interactions were generally ad hoc encounters, or reactive responses to perceived problems. Reflecting on these issues, members argued that limiting their potentially time consuming interactions with families was necessary in order to fulfil other work demands. Thus, the group's early discussions raised important concerns related to the staff's capacity to support family members in a manner consistent with a palliative approach to care. Subsequently, ARG members agreed that it was important to further explore these issues by investigating the perspectives of family care givers.

Action cycle 1

In action cycle 1, the ARG developed an action plan with the assistance of SA, to conduct a series of semi-structured interviews with family members of residents. The ARG members were closely involved in determining the content of the interview questions, which were intended to elicit family members' understandings of dementia, their experience of care processes, and having a relative resident on the DSU. The first author (SA) developed a draft interview schedule based on the ARG discussions and the group members reviewed the questions and provided feedback. Interviews were conducted with ten family members by SA. Findings from the interviews, subsequent to a first level analysis being undertaken by SA, were returned to the ARG to provoke their critical reflection on the issues raised.

The first level analysis of the interview data highlighted that family care givers had limited understandings about dementia, its progression, and how the DSU functioned. Moreover, the interview data provided poignant insights into family members' perceptions of ad hoc encounters by staff with them. Some held the impression that nursing and care staff had little desire to enter into a dialogue about care issues. Most family care givers did not consider that they were integral in a care-giving partnership.

Action research group reflections Group members reflected on the thematic analysis of the interview data, which provided rich ground for critical discussion. Through their meetings the group members worked to make sense of the issues raised by family members. Reflecting on the issues raised in the data, ARG members initially reiterated concerns about the implications of heavy workloads and short staffing. For example, one member Heather (RN), asserted that these circumstances had a profound impact on, 'time spent ... talking with and listening' to family care givers. Another member, Judy (RN), stated somewhat defensively: 'We can't explain it all [what's going on with care], we don't have the time!'

Yet, as the ARG members' critical engagement evolved, it became increasingly apparent that prioritizing task-based routines had the effect of circumventing interactions with family care givers. It became evident that in general, staff failed to address important information and consultation needs of family members. Judy shared a critical insight that captured this realization when she noted: 'I suppose they [family] are excluded from care.' Such insights challenged taken for granted assumptions about their practice. It highlighted an imperative to prioritize making information available to families about what one ARG member noted as: 'What [to expect] as the disease [dementia] progresses and what to expect when going to a dementia specific area'. However, at this stage the ARG discussions also revealed a lack of capacity within the organization to support this agenda. Thus, the group progressed to a second action cycle with an agreed position to develop a dementia information package for family members.

Stage 2: Emerging empowerment

Action cycle 2

In action cycle 2, group members worked to develop a plan of action through which they located various information resources related to dementia and reviewed these to develop a dementia information package. The resultant package included a booklet entitled 'Information for family and friends of people with severe and end stage dementia' (Palliative Care Dementia Interface: Enhancing Community Capacity Project, 2006), as well as a fact sheet containing information about the operation and characteristics of the DSU developed by two care staff members of the ARG. An evaluation form was also developed which sought feedback about the usefulness of the information package (Andrews *et al.*, 2009).

Action research group reflections The group members' reflections on action cycle 2 indicated growing recognition of the value of collaboration and the importance of sharing information and expertise. ARG members also shared renewed appreciation for the complexities of their job; for example, Elizabeth (PCA) conceded that prior to the study she had rarely considered, or discussed with her colleagues, the unique set of skills and knowledge she possessed. She stated: 'You don't really think about it, it's your job.' Catherine (PCA) agreed, adding that before the project she would not have conceived of developing an information resource for families; however, her participation had 'opened [her] eyes', about her ability as a care worker to contribute to improving care.

Stage 3: Reconfiguring practices

Action cycle 3

In action cycle 3 the ARG focused on planning and taking action to distribute the information packages to all family members of residents on the DSU. In total, the dementia information packages were distributed to 25 family members of residents, representing 89% of family care givers on the unit. Twenty-one of these family members returned evaluation forms, the results of which have been presented elsewhere (Andrews *et al.*, 2009). During this stage the group functioned largely independently of SA, with the exception of meeting to report their progress and discuss any concerns. By continuing to meet with the ARG members, the researcher was able to systematically document implementation activities and variations. During these meetings SA also adopted the role of a critical friend, asking questions of group members which encouraged them to continue to challenge their practices and personal assumptions.

Action research group reflections The ARG met three times after the completion of action cycle 3. Their initial reflections highlighted the central role played by the two PCAs (Catherine and Elizabeth) in leading the action. Judy (RN) explained that the nursing staff in the ARG supported Catherine and Elizabeth to take time out of their daily care routines to approach family members. She stated that this sort of team approach was highly successful in contacting all family members on the unit and providing them with an information package.

Group members discussed the positive changes in families' responses to staff and other residents after receiving the information packs. Catherine (PCA) explained how after personally approaching family members with the information, they had seized opportunities to engage: 'They are more responsive and they are more friendly.' During a subsequent meeting, care workers Catherine and Elizabeth reflected on how prior to the changes arising from the project, their interactions with families had been limited. Catherine reported how, prior to the research: 'We were never allowed to talk to family about things like this [referring to information about dementia in the DSU] . . . we always had to say, "look we'll just take you to the RN". We couldn't make a comment; it was just one of their [nursing staff] laws . . . just one of their guidelines'. Both Catherine and Elizabeth reported how they generally had avoided interaction with family care givers for fear of saying the wrong thing. Recognizing the effects of these conditions on their relations with family care givers, Catherine stated: 'I'm sure they [family] always felt like you were fobbing them off.' In the context where these staff had no prior opportunity to critically interrogate their practices, both care workers recognized that the situation was, as Elizabeth noted, 'Just something that we are accustomed to, it's normal'.

In a later meeting, Anne (RN) acknowledged that care workers on the unit generally 'weren't allowed' to discuss care issues with family members. Interestingly, this discussion represented the first occasion of an explicit acknowledgement by a nursing staff member of hierarchical power relations in silencing care workers in the dealing with family members. Such acknowledgment was significant as it led Catherine and Elizabeth to share with the group their new found confidence to approach family members to discuss care issues, knowing that they had back-up from more senior nursing staff. Catherine reported feeling: 'More comfortable in approaching [family care givers] and being out on the floor [in the unit] amongst them … I feel more at ease and more confident with what I say.'

Discussion

The findings of this study highlight the complex operation of power relations within the DSU and the action research process itself. At its early stages this was essentially a researcher-driven project; clearly a tension in the context of a research approach where the goal is empowerment of participants. Acknowledging the asymmetrical power relations between the researcher and ARG members at the outset of the project and acting to address these was crucial in establishing conditions that would support participant ownership of the research. However, the researchers were also aware of the hierarchical staffing arrangements that characterize aged care settings, and that the research site was no exception. Therefore, it was important for the researcher to direct the group to set up ground rules that would support each member to have an equal opportunity to contribute to the discussions. Gore (1992) explains that the exercise of power in an attempt to help others exercise power takes account of the micro dynamics of the operation of power in the given setting. From this perspective the researcher's engagement during the early stages of the project can be understood as an exercise of power to produce what might be referred to as a 'communicative space' (Kemmis, 2001: 103). The effects of this exercise of power produced a context where staff could engage in more democratic dialogic encounters, both with the researcher and with each other.

Through their early discussions, the ARG members revealed that organizational conditions profoundly shaped practice in ways that were reactive and essentially task-oriented. Action research group member accounts, which highlighted the inevitability and necessity of highly routine care, reflected the taken-for-granted nature of these practices. Returning the family interview data to the ARG was a powerful activity to stimulate the members' critical reflection on how they interacted with families. The interview data highlighted how the exercise of power by staff to avoid interactions with family, and hence minimize disruption to their routines, resulted in a subjugation of family members as key stakeholders in care processes. Given that a palliative approach to care relies on communication, support for, and collaboration with family members

(ADoHA, 2006), these circumstances highlight how the unwitting exercise of power by aged care staff can undermine best practice in this area.

Returning the interview data gathered from family members to ARG members was also an important activity in developing egalitarian relationships with the ARG members through the research process. The sharing of data reflected a negotiation of power between the researcher and participants, such that the researchers did not have a final say in the data interpretation. Rather, meaning was ascribed through a process that Lather (1991: 57) refers to as 'collaborative theorizing' between the participants and the researcher.

Through their critical engagement the ARG members began to recognize their own culpability in sustaining an unsupportive environment for family members. With this realization they began to conceive of family members' sense of exclusion, their lack of knowledge about dementia and the DSU as problems in which they shared responsibility. These critical insights in turn created an impetus for change, prompting the development of the dementia information package (action cycle 2). This action can be understood as strategic intervention by the group to disrupt their previous passive positions in response to family members' information needs. It can also be understood as an exercise of power by these staff to 'expand the boundaries' (Gaventa and Cornwell, 2001: 74) of their practice beyond historically constructed task-based roles. The empowering intent of critical action research was evident in the group's reflections (action cycle 2), which highlighted their growing awareness of themselves as active agents (Heron and Reason, 2001: 145) capable of interrogating their own understandings and producing critically informed knowledge.

Reflecting Foucault's (1977) knowledge/power nexus, the generation of critical knowledge opened up the possibilities for the ARG members to exercise power through their daily practices to improve the provision of a palliative approach to care. For example, in action cycle 3, ARG members' efforts to blur their role boundaries, such that the PCAs (Catherine and Elizabeth) were supported by the nursing staff in the ARG to personally approach family members, demonstrated a reconfiguration of power relations between staff to disrupt their historically hierarchical roles. The group members' reflections also suggested that prior to the study, hierarchal staff relations were part of what from a Foucault (1988) perspective could be deemed their most familiar landscape. The invisibility of these power relations was a key obstacle to the development of care practices that better reflected a palliative approach. However, it was only when the ARG took action to practice differently, and subsequently reflect on the effects (at the completion of action cycle 3), that the full implications of their historical ways of working were revealed. The reconfiguring of relations amongst the ARG members highlights how the productive features of power (Foucault, 1977: 119) can be harnessed to promote more equitable and meaningful relations between both staff themselves and staff and family members.

Finally, the growing independence of the ARG members as they progressed through the project also reflects a reconfiguration of power relations between the participants and researchers. As the group members' sustained engagement in critical dialogues exposed their own capacities to take action and their skills in research grew, the group members functioned more independently in the role of co-researchers (Heron and Reason, 2001).

Concluding remarks

In this chapter we have highlighted the complex operation of power relations in an aged care facility and the ways in which the unwitting exercise of power by aged care staff can undermine the development of collaborative relationships with family members of people with dementia. We have also discussed how power relations implicit in the action research process itself need to be acknowledged and addressed. With a critical awareness of how power relations shape the action research endeavour, participants can arrive at a critique of their situation and reconfigure how they exercise power in their everyday practice to produce more equitable and productive relationships with family members.

Acknowledgements

The authors wish to acknowledge the financial support provided by Southern Cross Care (Tas.) Inc. and the University of Tasmania to conduct this study.

References

Australian Bureau of Statistics (ABS) (2008) *Population Projections, Australia (3222.0)—2006 to 2010*. Canberra: Australian Bureau of Statistics. Available at: http://www.abs.gov.au/Ausstats/abs@.nsf/mf/3222.0.

Australian Institute of Health and Welfare (AIHW) (2010) *Residential Aged Care in Australia 2008–09: A Statistical Overview*. Canberra: Australian Institute of Health and Welfare. Available at: http://www.aihw.gov.au/WorkArea/DownloadAsset.aspx?id=6442472719.

Andrews, S., McInerney, F., and Robinson, A. (2009) Realizing a Palliative Approach in Dementia Care: Strategies to Facilitate Aged Care Staff Engagement in Evidence-Based Practice. *International Psychogeriatrics*, 21: S64–8.

Andrews, S., Lea, E., Haines, T., et al. (2012) Reducing Staff Isolation and Developing Evidence-Informed Practice in the Aged Care Environment through an Action Research Approach to Falls Prevention. *Advances in Nursing Science*, **35**(1): 3–13.

Angus, J. and Nay, R. (2003) The Paradox of the Aged Care Act 1997: The Marginalisation of Nursing Discourse. *Nursing Inquiry*, 10(2): 130–8.

Australian Department of Health and Ageing (ADoHA) (2006) *Guidelines for a Palliative Approach in Residential Aged Care, Enhanced Version*. Canberra: Australian Department of Health and Ageing.

Forbes, S., Bern-Klug, M., and Gessert, C. (2000) End of Life Decision Making for Nursing Home Residents with Dementia. *Journal of Nursing Scholarship*, 32(3): 251–8.

Foucault, M. (1977) Two Lectures. In: C. Gordon (ed.), *Power/Knowledge: Selected Interviews 1972-1977*, pp. 78–107. London: The Harvester Press.

Foucault, M. (1988) Truth, Power, Self: An Interview with Michel Foucault. In: L. Martin, H. Gytman, and P. Hutton (eds), *Technologies of the Self: A Seminar with Michel Foucault*, pp. 9–15. Amherst: The University of Massachusetts Press.

Froggatt, K., Wilson, D., Justice, C., et al. (2006) End of Life Care in Long Term Care Settings for Older People: A Literature Review. *International Journal of Older People Nursing*, 1(1): 45–50.

Gaventa, J. and Cornwell, A. (2001) Power and Knowledge. In: P. Reason and H. Bradbury (eds), *Handbook of Action Research*, pp. 71–82. London: Sage Publications.

Gore, J. (1992) What We Can Do for You! What Can 'We' Do for 'You'? Struggling over Empowerment in Critical and Feminist Pedagogy. In: C. Luke and J. Gore (eds), *Feminisms and Critical Pedagogy*, pp. 54–73. New York: Routledge.

Haesler, E., Bauer, M., and Nay, R. (2010) Recent Evidence on the Development and Maintenance of Constructive Staff-Family Relationships in the Care of Older People— A Report on a Systematic Review Update. *International Journal of Evidence-Based Healthcare*, **8**(2): 45–74.

Heron, J. and Reason, P. (2001) The Practice of Co-Operative Inquiry: Research 'With' Rather and 'On' People'. In: P. Reason and H. Bradbury (eds), *Handbook of Action Research*, pp. 144–54. London: Sage Publications.

Hockley, J. (2002) Organizational Structures for Enhancing Standards of Palliative Care. In: J. Hockley and D. Clark (eds) *Palliative Care for Older People in Care Homes*, pp. 165–81. Buckingham: Open University Press.

Jervis, L. (2002) Working in and Around the 'Chain of Command': Power Relations among Nursing Staff in an Urban Nursing Home. *Nursing Inquiry*, **9**(1): 12–23.

Kemmis, S. (2001) Exploring the Relevance of Critical Theory for Action Research: Emancipatory Action Research in the Footsteps of JurgenHabermas. In: P. Reason and H. Bradbury (eds), *Handbook of Action Research*, pp. 94–105. London: Sage Publications.

Kincheloe, J. and McLaren, P. (2008) Rethinking Critical Theory and Research. In: N.K. Denzin and Y.S. Lincoln (eds), *Handbook of Qualitative Research*, 3rd edn, pp. 403–56. Thousand Oaks: Sage Publications.

Knapp, M., Comas-Herrera, A., Somani, A., and Banerjee, S. (2007) *Dementia:Iinternational Comparisons*. King's College London: Personal Social Services Research Unit, London School of Economics and Political Science and the Institute of Psychiatry. Available free: www.pssru.ac.uk.

Koch, T. And Kralik, D. (2006) *Participatory Action Research in Health Care*. Oxford: Blackwell Publishing.

Lather, P. (1991) *Getting Smart: Feminist Research and Pedagogy with/in the Postmodern*. New York: Routledge.

Mason, R. and Boutilier, M. (1996) The Challenge of Genuine Power Sharing in Participatory Research: The Gap between Theory and Practice. *Canadian Journal of Community Mental Health*, 15(2): 145–52.

Mitchell, S., Teno, J., Kiely, D., et al. (2009) The Clinical Course of Advanced Dementia. *The New England Journal of Medicine*, 361(16): 1529–38.

Palliative Care Dementia Interface: Enhancing Community Capacity Project (2006) *Information for Family and Friends of People with Severe and End Stage Dementia*. Penrith, New South Wales: University of Western Sydney. Available from: http://www.uws.edu.au/__data/ assets/pdf_file/0008/7100/Dementia_Booklet_Final2011_PDFfor_web.pdf (accessed 30 October 2011).

Robinson, A. (1995) Transformative 'Cultural Shifts' In Nursing: Participatory Action Research and the 'Project Of Possibility'. *Nursing Inquiry*, 2(2): 65–74.

Street, A. and Robinson, A. (1995) Advanced Clinical Roles: Investigating Dilemmas and Changing Practice through Action Research. *Journal of Clinical Nursing*, 4(6): 349–57.

Chapter 12

Issues of diversity: participatory action research with indigenous peoples

Kevin Brazil

Participatory action research (PAR) has been identified as a form of inquiry well suited for indigenous peoples and communities (Bennett, 2004). Rooted in social justice, PAR typically combines the agenda of research, education, and social action with the intent to facilitate conditions for both individual and community change. Bennett (2004) identifies three types of change that could be anticipated through the PAR process: development of critical consciousness of both researcher and participants; improvement of the lives of those involved in the research process; and transformation of social structure and relationships. It is these aspects of PAR that have promoted its role as a mode of inquiry with indigenous peoples whose needs have not been addressed using the traditional Western research approach. In this chapter, the term 'Western' will be used to describe a world-view that is a product of the development of European culture. It represents knowledge, systems, rules, and values characteristically from Europe and the Western hemisphere (Ermine *et al.*, 2004).

This chapter will consider the relevance of the PAR approach with indigenous peoples and communities as it relates to a palliative care research project conducted in Canada. For many, the terms 'indigenous', 'aboriginal', 'First Nations', 'native', and 'Indian' are used interchangeably with limited appreciation of the meaning behind each expression. In Canada the term 'aboriginal' is commonly used to refer to First Nations, Métis, and Inuit peoples collectively. However, the criticism has been made that the word 'aboriginal' is a legal and social construction of the state and is associated with oppression (Chow, 2007). In subscribing to a critical PAR approach, the term 'indigenous' will be used to refer to the original peoples of Canada.

As part of this review, the historical relationship between Western oriented research and indigenous peoples in Canada will be described, and the promise and challenge of the PAR approach as a critical, anti-oppressive response to the conventional research approach will be examined. Finally, work on a palliative care research project I have undertaken with colleagues using a PAR framework, will be described. I acknowledge that this chapter is written 'outside' the indigenous community but reflects collaborative work with indigenous communities.

Characteristics of indigenous individuals and communities in Canada

In 2001, just over 1.3 million Canadians reported that their ancestors belonged to at least one of the indigenous communities recognized by Canada's Constitution, namely: First Nations, Métis, and Inuit people (Aboriginal Affairs and Northern Development Canada, 2012). While a great deal of diversity exists among the different indigenous groups across Canada, they share many experiences. Indigenous people in Canada do not share the same quality of life as the general population. They have higher unemployment, lower levels of education, and higher levels of poverty (Statistics Canada, 2009). From a health perspective, indigenous peoples in Canada experience a disproportionate burden of co-morbid health problems relative to the general Canadian population (Assembly of First Nations, 2005).

End-of-life care has become a priority among indigenous peoples within Canada (Assembly of First Nations, 2005; National Aboriginal Health Organization, 2012a). Due to a growing population and higher mortality due to accidents and complications of chronic disease, the need to develop appropriate palliative care programmes has become urgent. Consistent with trends in an aging population, health status reports indicate that rates of chronic and terminal disease are increasing among the indigenous community (Adelson, 2005; MacMillan *et al.*, 2003). The existing research provides an incomplete picture of the palliative care needs in this community. On the basis of a review of the available literature conducted by Kelly and Minty (2007), several factors were identified regarding end-of-life care in indigenous communities. These included: tensions between individual care decisions and family and community values; cultural beliefs and practices; and geographic isolation and its effects on medical resources. A significant barrier to indigenous communities in accessing palliative care is the absence of federal government funding. The Federal Government First Nations and Inuit Health Branch, which is responsible for the provision of a limited range of health services on reserves, does not presently fund palliative care, nor do clear policies exist regarding returning patients to their home communities when they are expected to die (Hotson *et al.*, 2004). The implications are that indigenous peoples, living in reserves in Canada, must develop palliative care programmes without government funding.

Given the identified barriers and the diversity of cultural beliefs and practices present among the indigenous peoples and communities located in Canada, knowledge generated by research may inform indigenous communities on the best approaches for providing palliative care. The understanding of indigenous peoples at an individual, family, and community level is a requisite for all research endeavors.

The historical relationship between research and indigenous peoples and communities

There is a general consensus among indigenous people that they have been 'researched to death' by academics and governments (Smith, 2001; Wilson, 2008). There exists an abundance of literature by non-indigenous academics writing about indigenous peoples from a Western perspective. Linda Tuhiwai Smith (2001) presented a critique of the Western concept of research that is practiced by mainstream academics. Research, argues Smith, has been integrated within European colonialism and as a consequence has been implicated in the worst excesses of colonialism and is a remembered history for many of the indigenous peoples.

In recent years, anti-oppressive scholars have argued that the standard researcher initiated approach that has traditionally driven the research process profits only the researcher, leaving little or no benefit to indigenous peoples and communities (Brown and Strega, 2005). The literature contains a plethora of recurring grievousness about the traditional research process (Bennett, 2004; Smith, 2001). As a response to how research has previously been conducted with indigenous peoples and communities, a number of indigenous organizations have asserted expectations on the values by which research should be conducted with indigenous peoples and communities. The development of the principles 'ownership, control, access, and possession' (OCAP) (Box 12.1), is recognized by many indigenous communities and organizations, and is an example of indigenous assertion on the determination of research concerning indigenous communities (Schnarch, 2004).

Ownership, control, access, and possession has served to enhance capacity building in indigenous research by bringing the concepts of ownership and control to the attention of communities (Schnarch, 2004). It has also furthered: the development of community-based research guidelines and agreements; how research ethics boards are to conduct ethical reviews of indigenous-related research; how community-based research information is accessed; and how palliative care research is conducted.

Box 12.1 Principles of ownership, control, access, possession.

- Ownership: Refers to the relationship of a First Nations community to its cultural knowledge/data/information. A community or group owns information collectively in the same way that an individual owns their personal information.

- Control: First Nations peoples, their communities, and representative bodies are within their rights in seeking to control all aspects of research and information management processes which impact them.

- Access: First Nations peoples must have access to information and data about themselves and their communities, and manage and make decisions regarding access to their collective information.

- Possession: Refers to the mechanism by which ownership (of data) can be asserted and protected

Data from Schnarch, B. (2004), Ownership, control, access, and possession (OCAP) or self-determination applied to research: a critical analysis of contemporary First Nations research and some options for First Nations communities. *Journal of Aboriginal Health*, **1**(1): 80–95.

In response to indigenous concerns on the practice of research, national organizations that fund Canadian research have developed ethical guidelines on how researchers should engage indigenous peoples and communities in the research process (Canadian Institutes of Health Research, 2010). In keeping with the OCAP principles, these ethical guidelines specify that researchers consult with the community, give community members the opportunity to be involved in all stages of the research, ensure ongoing communication with the community, and support education and training to build research capacity in the community. Ethical guidelines for researchers are needed to ensure that ethical principles are understood within the context of aboriginal concepts, such as sacred space and traditional knowledge. This may mean that ethical principles familiar to a researcher, such as autonomy, beneficence, and justice, would need to be adjusted to harmonize with the values and beliefs of indigenous peoples and communities.

The meaning of 'ethical space'

Despite the efforts of many people to create an ethic in research that changes the involvement of indigenous peoples, the issue of unequal relations between Western and indigenous knowledge systems still remains (Ermine *et al.*, 2004). Intrinsic within this relationship is a conflict of knowledge systems. The knowledge systems, rules, and values that make up the Western world-view have been critiqued by indigenous scholars as lacking the concepts by which the experience and reality of indigenous culture can be understood (Wilson, 2008). Consequently, indigenous knowledge systems are said to occupy a marginal position in relation to Western knowledge (Ermine *et al.*, 2004).

Indigenous and anti-oppressive scholars have identified the importance of developing an approach that promotes the co-creating of models of learning that bridge these two world-views. Reflecting this view, Willie Ermine (2004; 2007) has introduced the notion of 'ethical space' to describe the intersection of when the Western knowledge system meets the indigenous world-view. Building on Roger Poole's (1972) concept of ethical space, in his book, *Towards Deep Subjectivity*, Ermine applies the notion of ethical space to describe the space between the indigenous and Western cultures, and knowledge. These two knowledge systems hold distinct historical, political, linguistic, cultural, and economic realities (Ermine, 2004; 2007).

To Ermine, the intersection of where these two worlds meet represents an opportunity in which meaningful and authentic dialogue between individuals from these two worlds can take place, enabling research to engage in different knowledge systems; thus, providing the potential of co-creating a new way of learning. According to Ermine, a fundamental requirement for meaningful engagement is to acknowledge the existence of an ethical space between the two world-views. Ethical space cannot exist without this affirmation (Ermine, 2004; 2007).

Recognizing this ethical space contributes to facilitating a dialogue between university-based, Western-oriented researchers and indigenous communities on the intentions, values, and assumptions in the research process. Authentic dialogue can avoid the false dichotomy between Western and indigenous knowledge. Rather, a dialogue within ethical space can facilitate acceptance of differences between these systems as well as finding similarities between the two points of view (Ermine, 2004; 2007). An important dimension to ethical space is the participants' individual emancipation from belief systems that have suppressed their awareness of how systems of thought have shaped their lives, and their personal capacity for change and engaging in social transformation (Ermine, 2004; 2007). Dialogue within an ethical space can facilitate cross-cultural engagement, which can lead to research agreement between researchers and indigenous communities on questions such as: Whose research is it? Who owns it? Who will benefit from it? Who will carry it out? How will the results be shared? (Smith, 2001).

The application of participatory action research

A PAR approach that includes a critical or emancipatory perspective is a mode of inquiry (see Chapter 2) that resonates with Ermine's description of ethical space, where different groups can come together and co-develop a vision and purpose for a research project. The emancipatory aspect of PAR aims to assist those engaged in the research, researchers, and community members alike, to develop a critical under-standing of their situation. According to Freire (1970), emancipation requires a proc-ess of conscientization, in which individuals develop an awareness of the social, cultural, and political forces that shape their lives as well as their own capacity to respond to those forces. Ethical space is a location that can facilitate Freire's notion of critical consciousness.

A key element of PAR is that it takes a critical theory approach; this means that it recognizes and addresses the political and social structures that can empower and oppress certain groups. Critical theory accepts the fact of historical oppression. For indigenous people in Canada, PAR includes a critique on the impact of colonization and marginalization (Hoare *et al.*, 1993). This critical perspective located within PAR is what has promoted its acceptance with indigenous communities. Its methods and processes promote empowerment, inclusivity, and respect. Most importantly, this approach serves to deconstruct the Western research paradigm and is inclusive toward an indigenous understanding of knowledge.

While PAR holds promise as a research approach, it is also an approach that holds no clear guidelines on how it should be implemented (Bennett, 2004). While this rep-resents a strength, whereby the process can be easily adapted to suit the context, at the same time this can challenge participants on what represents PAR. The author's expe-rience of PAR in a palliative care research project will be used as an illustrative example on the considerations that can transpire in a PAR research approach with indigenous communities.

In 2010, the author, with colleague Mary Lou Kelley (see Chapter 4) were the recipi-ents of funding from the Canadian Institutes of Health Research to conduct a five-year research project, 'Improving end-of- life care in First Nations communities: Generating a theory of change to guide program and policy development'. The overall goal of this intervention is to build on the strengths and resources in four indigenous communi-ties to improve end-of-life care (Prince and Kelley, 2010). Four indigenous communi-ties agreed to participate in this project: Naotkamegwanning First Nation, Fort William First Nation, Six Nations of the Grand River Territory, and Peguis First Nation.

Partnering in all phases of research is a common recommendation for successful work with indigenous communities and was a founding principle for this project. The four communities agreed to participate in the project during the development stages, during which the research plan was developed through a dialogue among representatives of the partnering communities. Following recommendations from their local healthcare providers, the chiefs of the involved communities reviewed the plan and consented to participate in the project. This process ensured that the proposed research represented a topic of mutual interest representing local community priorities (Fletcher, 2003; LaVeaux and Christopher, 2009). By the time the project was launched, following a successful peer review process, each community had developed a project advisory committee that included community members. Each committee has the role of overseeing all aspects of the research process within their community, assisting in community engagement, identifying the appropriate participants, reviewing preliminary data interpretation, identifying community interventions, and developing an inclusive dissemination plan. The presence of the community advisory committees ensures that community participation is a focal point rather than a minor element of the research process and also that the principles of OCAP are active in the project (Fletcher, 2003).

An element of PAR is the integration of knowledge sharing within the partnership process. In this project, members of the project advisory committee were offered training on PAR, research ethics, and the requirement of rigour for the research. Likewise, the researchers were socialized by community partners on the characteristics of the communities, including their values and customs. This exchange represented a co-learning of the respective worlds occupied by project participants. The underlying principle of the co-learning was that the project participants understand the forces that drove individual actions, thereby facilitating a greater opportunity for authentic interaction among participants (Fletcher, 2003; LaVeaux and Christopher, 2009).

A community facilitator was hired by each community project advisory committee to lead local implementation of the project. With guidance from the research team, these individuals facilitate community engagement, and identify and assess community interventions. Regional, provincial, and national partnerships have also been developed to support the four communities in developing their community interventions.

In keeping with a PAR approach, initial project activities have included community engagement and community assessment specific to developing palliative care within each community. Working with the community advisory committees, these activities have generated community awareness of the project as well as information for the development of community-specific palliative care interventions. These initial project activities, which have generated community engagement in the project, have affirmed the fact that no two communities are the same and that a respect for the uniqueness of each community and research situation is required (Fletcher, 2003; LaVeaux and Christopher, 2009).

Our experience showed that it is important to allow sufficient time for each community to become involved in a project. Timeframes for successful community engagement are dependent on the character of the community. As has been recommended by others (Fletcher, 2003; LaVeaux and Christopher, 2009), time should be allocated for cultural differences that may make communication slower than researchers would prefer or anticipate. Researchers must allow the community to establish the sequence and timing of activities (Fletcher, 2003). It is also important that the researcher/s may have to learn about their own approach to research within such a project.

Researchers must also recognize that communities are complex, with individuals and groups representing different interests and values, or holding different levels of influence or power. For example, not all people in a community may want to participate in PAR or participation may be sporadic. Some individuals in the community may be suspicious of the benefits to the community (Bennett, 2004). Researchers must navigate these relationships, while taking care not to promote false expectations on the benefits of the research nor reinforce unequal power relations in the community (Bennett, 2004).

Parallel to the assertion and control of research, as well as the recognition of PAR as a relevant mode of research, there has also been development of 'insider research' within the indigenous communities; a term that describes research conducted by indigenous researchers (Ermine *et al.*, 2004). 'Outsider research' has been used to describe non-aboriginal researchers who characterize much of the history of research on indigenous people. The growth of indigenous researchers has promoted the emergence of research paradigms that are rooted in an indigenous world-view. These trends represent a movement by indigenous communities no longer to act as passive recipients of research activities. In our project eight members of the research team are of indigenous heritage, which helped to ensure that the project adheres to culturally appropriate principles and an indigenous world-view. Acknowledging the importance of insider-based research, student training targeting indigenous students is a major component to the project, furthering the capacity for indigenous-directed research practice.

While there is no single approach to conducting PAR, working with indigenous communities introduces additional considerations that researchers need to understand. Sensitivity to these considerations promotes more sustainable impacts from the research for the participating communities. These considerations highlight that PAR is an approach that requires researchers to be open and receptive as well as flexible in responding to the situations they may encounter.

Conclusion

Research in indigenous communities requires that attention be paid to the historical developments that have led these communities to where they are today. This chapter has attempted to outline the promise and challenge of PAR as a principal research approach with indigenous peoples and communities. It has also outlined the unique considerations that have been identified for PAR researchers who pursue research with indigenous communities.

Acknowledgement

The author would like to thank the peoples of the communities of Naotkamegwanning First Nation, Fort William First Nation, Peguis First Nation, and Six Nations of the

Grand River Territory for extending their welcome and trust to me. The expression of this chapter is inspired by the relationships between me and various members of these communities. This chapter is a token of thanks for the lessons I have been taught.

References

Aboriginal Affairs and Northern Development Canada (2012) *Aboriginal Peoples and Communities*. Available at: http://www.aadnc-aandc.gc.ca/eng/1100100013785/1304467449155 (accessed 2 February 2012).

Adelson, N. (2005) The Embodiment of Inequality: Health disparities in Aboriginal Canada. *Canadian Journal of Public Health*, **96**: 45–60.

Assembly of First Nations (2005) *First Nations Action Plan on Continuing Care*. Available at: http://64.26.129.156/cmslib/general/CCAP.pdf (accessed 30 January 2012).

Bennett, M. (2004) A Review of the Literature on the Benefits and Drawbacks of Participatory Action Research. *First Peoples Child & Family Review*, 1(1): 19–32.

Brown, L. and Strega, S. (2005) *Research as Resistance Critical, Indigenous, and Anti-oppressive Approaches*. Toronto: Canadian Scholars' Press.

Canadian Institutes of Health Research (CIHR) (2010) *Canadian Institutes of Health Research, Natural Sciences and Engineering Research Council of Canada and Social Sciences and Humanities Research Council of Canada, Tri-Council Policy Statement: Ethical Conduct for Research Involving Humans*. Available at: http://www.pre.ethics.gc.ca/pdf/eng/tcps2/TCPS_2_FINAL_Web.pdf (accessed January 2012).

Chow W. (2007) *Three-Partner Dancing: Placing Participatory Action Research Theory into Practice with an Indigenous, Racialized and Academic Space*. Available at: https://dspace.library.uvic.ca:8443/handle/1828/190 (accessed 2 February 2012).

Ermine, W. (2004) *Ethical Space: Transforming Relations*. Paper delivered at University of Saskatchewan Indigenous Knowledge Symposium: Saskatoon, SK, May 2004.

Ermine, W. (2007) The Ethical Space of Engagement. *Indigenous Law Journal*, 6: 193–203.

Ermine, W., Sinclair, R., and Jeffery B. (2004) *The Ethics of Research Involving Indigenous People's Health Research Centre to the Interagency Advisory Panel on Research Ethics*. Saskatoon, SK: Indigenous People's Health Research Centre.

Fletcher, C. (2003) Community-Based Participatory Research Relationships with Aboriginal Communities in Canada: An Overview of Context and Process. *Pimatziwin: A Journal of Aboriginal and Indigenous Community Health*, **1**(1): 27–62.

Freire, P. (1970) *Pedagogy of the Oppressed*. New York: The Continuum Publishing Corporation.

Hoare, T., Levy, C., and Robinson, M.P. (1993) Participatory Action Research in Native Communities: Cultural Opportunities and Legal Implications. *The Canadian Journal of Native Studies*, **13**(1). Available at: http://www2.brandonu.ca/library/cjns/13.1/hoare.pdf (accessed 31 January 2012).

Hotson, K., Macdonald, S., and Martin, B. (2004) Understanding Death and Dying in Select First Nations Communities in Northern Manitoba: Issues of Culture and Remote Service Delivery in Palliative Care. *International Journal of Circumpolar Health*, 63(1): 25–38.

Kelly, L. and Minty, A. (2007) End of Life Issues for Aboriginal Patients. *Canadian Family Physician*, **53**: 1459–65.

LaVeaux, D. and Christopher, S. (2009) Contextualizing CBPR: Key Principles of CBPR Meet the Indigenous Research Context. *Pimatisiwin: A Journal of Aboriginal and Indigenous Community Health*, 7(1): 1–25.

MacMillan, H.L., Walsh, C.A., Jamieson, E., et al. with the Technical Advisory Committee of the Chiefs of Ontario (2003) The health of Ontario First Nations People. *Canadian Journal of Public Health*, 94(3): 168–72.

National Aboriginal Health Organization (NAHO) *Discussion Paper on End of Life/Palliative Care for Aboriginal Peoples*. Available at: http://www.naho.ca/documents/naho/french/pdf/re_briefs2.pdf (accessed 31 January 2012).

Poole, R. (1972) *Towards Deep Subjectivity*. London: The Penguin Press.

Prince, H. and Kelley, M.L. (2010) An Integrative Framework for Conducting Palliative Care Research with First Nations Communities. *Journal of Palliative Care*, **26**: 47–53.

Schnarch, B. (2004) Ownership, Control, Access, and Possession (OCAP) or Self-Determination Applied to Research: A Critical Analysis of Contemporary First Nations Research and Some Options for First Nations Communities. *Journal of Aboriginal Health*, 1(1): 80–95.

Smith, L.T. (2001) *Decolonizing Methodologies: Research and Indigenous Peoples*. London: Zed Books.

Statistics Canada, Canada Year Book (2009) *Aboriginal Peoples*. Available at: http://www41.statcan.gc.ca/2009/10000/cybac10000_000-eng.htm (accessed 2 February 2012).

Wilson, S. (2008) *Research is Ceremony: Indigenous Research Methods*. Nova Scotia: Fernwood Publishing.

Wilson, K. and Rosenburg, M. W. (2002) Exploring the Determinant of Health for First Nations People in Canada: Can Existing Frameworks Accommodate Traditional Activities? *Social Science and Medicine*, **55**(11): 2017–31.

Chapter 13

Gender perspectives in Austrian participatory research in palliative care for older people

Elisabeth Reitinger and Erich Lehner

Theoretical insights, empirical studies and research experience show that gender influences our lives from the very beginning to the very end. As a social category, gender gives structure to societies as well as imposing opportunities and constraints on people throughout the life course. In health and social research it is well acknowledged that there are influences and interconnections between gender, health, and ageing (Backes *et al.*, 2006; WHO, 2003). There has been increasing emphasis on gender and more recently within palliative care (Beyer, 2008; Reitinger and Lehner, 2009).

Social interactions and relationships that are crucial for caring as well as doing participatory research include personal involvement and gender interpretations. 'Doing gender' is a phenomenon that has been reflected on and discussed in detail in gender studies, feminist studies (Ribbens *et al.*, 1998), and critical men´s studies. However, within the context of participatory research in palliative care for older people, it is a new perspective of thinking and methodological approach.

In this chapter we will reflect gender perspectives in two ways. The first will highlight the way gender influences research projects, including ethical aspects. The second will focus on findings from two participatory research projects we conducted; the first, in collaboration with a long-term care setting for older people in Tirol, a province of Austria, during 2009–2011; the second, in a large long-term care provider in Vienna, Austria.

We start our discussion by exploring the conceptual and empirical background of palliative care for and with older people, a gender framework, and an outline of our methodological approach in relation to participatory research. The chapter finishes with a discussion that opens up considerations for further integration of gender into participatory research projects in palliative care for older people.

Conceptual and empirical background to our use of gender in participatory research

Talking about gender in participatory research requires an understanding of palliative care for older people as well as the conceptual basis of gender. To give an insight into how this intervention is undertaken we describe our methodological approach within participatory research.

Palliative care for older people

Living with old age has an impact on individuals, their families, friends, and society as a whole. The vulnerability that characterizes human beings becomes more obvious when care needs appear. Women and men in old age often live with different diseases that include limitations in mobility and the probability of developing dementia. Older people therefore rely on the help and care of others. Palliative care for older people has become acknowledged as an essential approach in end-of-life care especially in long-term care settings (Davies and Higginson, 2004; Heimerl, 2008; Heller *et al.*, 2003; Hockley and Clark, 2002).

Institutionalized long-term care settings have increased in importance as places of care as a result of changes in the provision of care in modern societies. Although a high percentage of care is still taken on by relatives informally, institutionalized long-term care (LTC) settings or nursing homes meet many care demands. Older people who go to live there are often confronted with dramatic changes: new living environments, loss of social relations, and the awareness that life will come to an end sooner rather than later (Heller *et al.*, 2003). These circumstances influence their overall bodily, cognitive, emotional, and social status. Families of residents living in LTC settings or nursing homes regularly have to deal with ambiguous feelings of relief and guilt and also have needs to be met (Reitinger, 2006). Palliative care as an approach offers insights, experiences, and practice that help in the care for older people and has been integrated in a number of LTC settings or nursing homes throughout different European countries and even worldwide (Froggatt *et al.*, 2009; 2011; Heller *et al.*, 2007; Kojer, 2009; Pleschberger, 2007).

However, the rationalization and economization in healthcare and social systems in Austria and other Western societies have taken their toll. Reduction of qualified staff and financial cutbacks weaken the resource base for the care of older people, including the impact on end-of-life care. Management of care institutions faces irresolvable conflicts when a user-driven higher demand in quantity and quality, alongside diversity of needs, is faced with fewer resources (Heimerl, 2006; Heller *et al.*, 2003; Reitinger, 2006). These conflicts, arising from a variety of imbalances between the public and the private sphere, lead to a general care deficit (Hochschild, 1995). Traditionally, the care of older people has been unpaid informal work in the home. However, the effect of the increasing status of paid work alongside the withdrawal of public funding has led to 'cold-modern' and 'postmodern' ways of providing care within society. The term 'cold-modern' (Hochschild, 1995) refers to care that is performed as a rational task organized in a practical and efficient way without showing emotion. Such care imposes maximum working hours, exploiting employees who can often be perceived by management as human capital.

Another contradiction within the day-to-day work of nursing homes is that the life worlds of the frail elderly and, indeed, staff working in nursing homes need to be of equal importance alongside structures of the organization(s) (Hockley, 2006). As institutions have to follow certain processes (such as efficiency and quality management), structures are built in order to monitor care. These circumstances, of course, influence the place of a palliative care culture for frail older people living and dying in these settings (Hockley, 2002; Reitinger, 2006; Small *et al.*, 2007).

Gender framework

In our research we follow a social constructionist approach where the sex-gender differentiation is fundamental: 'sex' refers to females´ and males' biological features, whereas 'gender' understands women and men in relation to the social impact of their sex. This gender concept enables a reflection about women and men without viewing them just as biologically determined. However, the question of the relationship between sex and gender still remains. If there is no determination of biology, and sex is not the basic ground for gender, can the body be perceived as something that exists before any social construction? Different positions have been formulated to answer this question. We are convinced that there is no relationship between sex and gender according to the principle of cause and effect. There is a constant interplay between both biology and gender (Schmitz, 2006).

To counter the distinction of sex and gender, West and Zimmerman (1987) in their concept of 'doing gender' represent gender identity as a permanent social construction process, which goes along with all human practice: 'Doing gender involves a complex of socially guided perceptual, interactional, and micro-political activities that cast particular pursuits as expressions of masculine and feminine "nature"' (West and Zimmerman, 1987: 126). It could be argued, therefore, that gender is on the one hand institutionalized, 'in structure, as well as being an aspect of individual character or personality' (Connell, 2000: 29).

In describing gender within our palliative care research with older people/LTC facilities, it is helpful to consider four dimensions (Lehner and Reitinger, 2008: 142), namely:

- Structure: at this level one asks, how are men and women participating? What roles and functions do they find themselves in, and what rules do they have to obey?
- Relationships and interaction: the leading question here is, how are gender relations (re)produced through daily face-to-face-interactions?
- Culture of an institution: this considers, what aspects of gender are dominant in a certain institution? how are people expected to act in relation to their gender?
- Personal identity: this asks, how are personal identities and individuals supported within this culture?

Participatory research—our journey explored

Based on experiences from two empirical studies, we present our approach to participatory research founded on core methodological elements of a trans-disciplinary (Reitinger, 2008) and qualitative paradigm alongside an understanding of research as intervention (Heintel, 2003; Krainer, 2006).

The central themes of the projects were 'gender aspects in long-term care' and 'ethical decisions in nursing homes' (Reitinger, 2008; Reitinger and Lehner, 2009). Both projects were conducted in Austria in collaboration with a total number of four nursing homes from different provider organizations.

Participatory research within a trans-disciplinary approach starts with listening, talking, and walking around. In collaboration with nursing home staff, discussion begins by sitting at a table with management to agree on the topics and forms of cooperation. This initiates a trustful relationship. This communication, importantly within and across boundaries, relies on appreciative interactions that establish meaningful social spaces. This reflects the principle of appreciative inquiry (as described in Chapter 6). Interviews, group discussions, and observation are common methods used during such an inquiry.

For the context of the research projects on 'gender in nursing homes' and 'ethical decisions' it was important to continuously reflect on the research process and find the connections and boundaries between content (gender, ethical decisions) and form (participatory approach). Following the German concept of participative intervention-research (Heintel, 2003, Krainer, 2006), opportunities for self-reflection were organized in order to fulfil the aims of both knowledge-production as well as bring about change within social systems. Questions and reflections initiated at the level of individual *and* social systems lead to changes in awareness and expertise that overcome the 'division of labour in scientific knowledge production' (Heintel, 2003: 23). Individual and organizational empowerment as well as emancipation can be formulated as leading principles of the research approach in use. It is based on the belief that professionals and also patients and relatives are experts of both their living and working situation. The questions asked by the researchers therefore aim at making explicit the often implicit knowledge, expertise, and experience. Another premise is that all persons and social systems participating in a research project can learn from each other and it is only through relationships that something new can emerge. This individual and collective learning does have emancipatory effects.

The principles just outlined above have parallels to participatory action research (PAR). Aiming at a 'collaborative, equitable partnership in all phases of the research' (Blair and Minkler, 2009: 653) both tactics intend to create appreciative relationships with those involved. The traditions of empowering, co-learning, and systems change within PAR accurately meet basic principles of the trans-disciplinary framework. Balancing research and action is essential.

Sampling in both projects started from a case study design (Yin, 1994). Collaboration with nursing homes of different providers working on diverse legal and structural backgrounds as well as varying organizational cultures were established. The research process then was an iterative one. From the very beginning, reflective sessions were included to ensure a better understanding of how we can successfully cooperate with our partners from the nursing homes, what questions make sense, and what issues were the most important threads to bear in mind throughout the project. In interviews and focus groups, stories and narratives were formulated by individuals or within the interdisciplinary team. Written and spoken words are one basis of interpretations. Observations of important social settings within the nursing homes, for example lunch-time or the lobby area, additional verbal and also non-verbal signs and processes contributed to the data base (Lamnek, 2005). Analyses of data were conducted individually through coding and categorizing as well as in discussion processes within the research teams.

Reflective sessions within the research team were undertaken. These helped to identify assumptions and formulate assessments of the current situation alongside new perspectives for further steps. Conflicts that flared up within the research team often mirrored tensions within the cooperating nursing homes and revealed critical issues. Talking about the often hidden issue of abuse in care situations (e.g. forcing a resident to have a wash) also led to conflicting positions within the research team. By discussing the different arguments, diverse ethical standpoints and moral values became obvious; this is turn mirrored difficulties that professionals were facing in the nursing homes.

Results and interpretations were then validated with practitioners in different settings. Gender or ethical issues that were identified as central to the care, at the same time affected organizational matters. These central issues were prepared for presentation in group discussions with management (Bohnsack, 2002). Presentations on different hierarchical levels involved a variety of perspectives and gave staff the opportunity for diversity in interpretation (Reitinger and Heimerl, 2008). Options for implementation of gender-sensitive care or ethical situation analyses were elaborated and led to a broader cultural awareness.

Challenges addressing gender in participatory research

We now share two specific challenges while undertaking our research. First, we highlight some of the ethical considerations encountered from a gender perspective when undertaking participatory research, including power dynamics and the issue of informed consent. Second, we will consider the gender issues in caring for frail older people within the field of palliative care.

'Doing gender' while undertaking participatory research: Ethical reflections

As participatory researchers seeking for collaboration we involve ourselves, our values, beliefs, knowledge, attitudes, and emotions with those who could be interested in such projects. As gendered beings, the influence of gendered interactions will be present throughout the research process. It begins with the question of who is a project leader, or the decision about the inclusion of men and women in the research team at the structural level. However, it becomes more complex when reflecting about the influence of gender in interview situations or group discussions. Processes of 'doing gender' and gendered aspects of different themes, for example emotions, task-orientation, relation-orientation, or coping with pain and bereavement, have to be observed simultaneously. As findings concerning patient-doctor communication indicate, the readiness of showing emotions, for example, depends on the gender of the medical doctor.

> Findings show that certain topics of discussion may be avoided in the different dyads. For example, male patients may find it difficult to talk to male doctors about emotional agendas, but raise them more frequently with female doctors. This is not surprising as women are stereotyped as being more emotional and hence the best people to deal with others' emotions.
> (Sandhu et al., 2009: 353)

Comparing doctor-patient relationships with researcher-participant relationships, this and other gender effects influence interview and workshop situations similarly. The reflections of our own research relationships with residents of the nursing home led us to propose that gender *did* have effects. Our research team comprised of a female and male researcher. As we reflected, some issues (e.g. sexual wishes) can only be formulated in a male-male dyad; on the other hand we observed that within a female-female dyad it is more likely that emotions are shown.

Other differences were noticeable. Within the participatory projects we conducted, practitioners had practical tasks to be doing within the setting, and were often keen to be 'told what to do'. This was in conflict with the researchers, whose role was to spend time reflecting and working out the broader issues together. Conflicts arose because of these differences and needed to be dealt with.

Power relations are often related to gender issues. Interpersonal conflicts may occur within the setting; these are often attributed to power, as already discussed; however, it may be more about gender without it being recognized. Furthermore, there are social constructions about what a good researcher has to do. In relation to practitioners from nursing homes it seems to be important as a researcher to retain a certain status as an expert. In this role as an expert, more power is deferred to the research partners concerning the research process.

Ethical questions of responsibility have to be reflected on a regular basis. This is not only necessary at the individual level but also at the team and organizational level. Hidden agendas that influence power dynamics have to be dealt with, such as the necessary collaboration between researchers within the hierarchical university system and management/staff working within the hierarchical care institutions system. For a good researcher or research team, a certain match is necessary for his/her/their career to engage in third-party funding to undertake research. On the other hand, research projects can also help collaborating institutions to legitimate their work and to show their innovative potential. High pressure and interdependence therefore lead to a complex interplay of power. As researchers, we depend on the interest, trust, and time of practitioners within the care instructions for collaboration. We have to take the necessary time to create a common understanding. But, at the same time professionals are in need of quick solutions and practical recommendations; for example how to support gender-sensitive care within an institution. In addition, as researchers, it is important to use an appreciative approach but at the same time share critical comments on what is going on (i.e. when in our view we uncovered a situation of abuse). Taking our research activities seriously in order to communicate openly runs the risk that practitioners quit their collaboration.

Concerning gender issues, questions about power relations have to be differentiated even more. Riley *et al.* (2003) explored the dynamics of subjectivity and power between researchers and those taking part in the study (the researched), and integrated the gender dimension in polyvocal narratives. One experience of a female PhD student conducting interviews with male managers supported findings from other feminist writers that 'the power dynamics of their research were not mapped out along an axis of researcher–researched (powerful–powerless) but on gendered dimensions of male–female (powerful–powerless)' (Riley *et al.*, 2003: 28). The act of silencing herself during the interviews and balancing harmonious social relationships produced a sense of powerlessness. At the same time, the situations produced a sexualized subject position where female youth and attractiveness balanced male knowledge and intelligence. Power dynamics gained in transparency by discussing different perspectives.

When doing participatory research in the field of palliative care for older people, ethical questions are part of everyday considerations. Aspects, such as changing the researcher–participant relationship into collaborative engagement, issues of informed consent, ethical approval, and ethical reflections, need special awareness. 'It is not possible to hide behind the research method when things get difficult. This means that an ethical way of being, which relates to human interrelationships, is likely to be more important than procedural ethical codes' (Burns, 2007: 161).

Informed consent aims at making sure that participants know what they agree to when participating in a research project, and that they decide voluntarily and understand the implications of what they are doing. Formal written agreements include information about the topics of the research project, the aims, and how the research will be undertaken and analysed. Anonymity and confidentiality are usually important parts of the agreement. Within participatory research, where the design of the whole project is in constant change and the full scope of the research activities are typically negotiated with participants, informed consent seems to be difficult. Due to the emergent and revolving character of PAR sometimes it is not possible to completely specify all steps that will develop at the beginning of the project. Within our project, for example, at the beginning we planned to have three different presentations of the results within each provider organization. Due to the interest of the practitioners this plan changed into a common presentation with reflection across the borders of the provider organizations. Ethical themes and issues were talked about there and then in an unexpected open atmosphere.

Another aspect that is vital in participatory research projects with palliative care for older people is the ethical question of listening to the voices that are often neglected, giving them a protective space and at the same time engaging in emancipatory questions at a structural or systemic level (Burns, 2007). Gender effects seem especially important. Opening up opportunities to communicate with older persons in nursing homes, and asking them very personal questions concerning their biography, their actual relationships, and the meaning of supporting relatives, means that issues can be addressed that often remain invisible or silent. This knowledge is important for gender-sensitive care. However, at the same time such knowledge does not enable change in the underlying structural and social aspects (i.e. the strongly gender-segregated and underpaid care work). Knowing about the gendered biography of a certain woman helps one understand her needs, but on its own does not change the organization in a way to give staff more time for each resident. The changes of gendered structures need to be supported at a political level as well.

Ethical questions also rise during analysis and interpretation of data. Being serious in validating interpretations in collaboration with practitioners gives opportunity for gender stereotypes to gain support. Critical perspectives formulated mainly by the researchers on the other hand might be challenged by those in practice and provoke resistance to change. Therefore we think that it is important to have the opportunity to have common interpretations between the research team as well as interpretations by the research team and the practitioners.

Gender dimensions in palliative care for older people

Concentrating on palliative care in LTC settings/nursing homes for frail older people in Austria, it is important to mention that these institutions can be described as female life worlds. A high percentage (70–90%) of the residents, professionals, relatives, informal care givers, and volunteers are women. This gender bias also plays an important role concerning the overall value of the whole sector of elderly care within society (Acker, 1992; Backes *et al.*, 2006; Beyer, 2008; Kreutzner, 2006; Reitinger and Lehner, 2009).

Care work has traditionally been, and still is, a female profession encompassing communication, physical care, and emotional labour, and is primarily engaged in meeting the needs of the residents. Building trustful relationships and appreciative communication are often implicit competencies that remain tacit in an interpretation of care work oriented mainly towards action and manual labour. Gender segregation of work that is connected with a devaluation of female competencies, together with the high physical, psychological, and emotional stress that characterize working in nursing homes, lead to the feeling of 'being wrung out' (James, 2009; Twigg, 2006). As Hochschild (1983) argues, emotional labour requires the competence to coordinate mind and feeling in such a way that the emotions of an individual carer can be withheld for the sake of being able to care for the needs and feelings of the client/s. Emotional labour, therefore, concerns the deep structure of personal identity.

We identified four areas of conflict in which gender became significant in our study. These encompassed: the individual situation of residents; carer interactions; family relationships; and, management. So first, gendered biographies play an essential role and have an impact on care situations. The ability to accept help and care, for example, correlates with life experiences. For some women it is not easy to accept help in their room when they have been used to managing a household for all of their life. However, for other women, they are glad and content to get the care and help. For some men it is difficult to accept the dependence on women for their care needs; yet others see care as women's work, so they have no problem in accepting it.

Second, nurses reported that female needs frequently appeared in the form of lament and complaint; whereas, men often expressed themselves with a combination of demand and accusation. Mostly it is difficult for female nurses to cope with these male demands. From the professional/carer aspect in our study, it seemed easier for male personnel to distance themselves from the challenging needs of residents.

Third, most relatives in contact with the resident in the home are females. Male residents usually receive care from their wives, while female residents mostly rely on the relationship with their children. We also found a difference in the regularity of the visits: male visitors did not visit so often, whereas female visitors showed more continuity.

Finally, management and administration play an essential role when looking at gender effects within an organization. Leading and running an institution like a home is still qualified as 'male'. This goes along with the observation that different languages are spoken. One is the emotional language of the nurses shaped by the experience of the relationship which is associated as female. On the other hand, there is the language of figures characterized by an economical thinking, attributed to men, alongside the male-dominated language of medicine. These languages represent important areas of care in the home. However, often there does not seem to be a link between them. These findings show important aspects when gender is reflected on through a PAR study within a nursing home caring for frail older people at the end of life.

Conclusion

In conclusion we would like to sum up the most important insights of our thoughts, experiences, and reflections with respect to existing knowledge and research evidence. The fact that we are gendered beings seems to be the essential starting point. Gender as a social construct has effects on individual, relational, and structural levels. Within participatory research projects in palliative care for older people, gender influences research interactions, decision making, and results. As we highlighted, ethical questions are interconnected with gender aspects in different ways. Power effects within participatory research, as well as in gender relations, should be reflected upon.

References

Acker, J. (1992) Gendering Organizational Theory. In: A. J. Mills and P. Tancred (eds), *Gendering Organizational Analysis*, pp. 248–60. Newbury Park: Sage.

Backes, G.M., Lasch, V., and Reimann, K. (2006) *Gender, Health and Ageing: European Perspectives on Life Course, Health Issues and Social Challenges*. Wiesbaden: VS-Verlag.

Beyer, S. (2008) *Frauen im Sterben: Gender und Palliative Care*. Freiburg: Lambertus.

Blair, T. and Minkler, M. (2009) Participatory Action Research with Older Adults: Key Principles in Practice. *Gerontologist*, **49**(5): 651–62.

Bohnsack, J. (2002) *Rekonstruktive Sozialforschung: Einführung in Qualitative Methoden*. Stuttgart: UTB.

Burns, D. (2007) Quality and Ethics in Systemic Action Research. In: D. Burns (ed.), *Systemic Action Research: A Strategy for Whole System Change*, pp. 155–71. Bristol: The Policy Press, Bristol.

Connell, R.W. (2000) *The Man and the Boys*. Berkely: University of California Press.

Davies, E. and Higginson, I. (2004) *Better Palliative Care for Older People*. Copenhagen: World Health Organization.

Froggatt, K., Davies, S., and Meyer, J. (2009) Research and Development in Care Homes: Setting the Scene. In: K. Froggatt, S. Davies, and J. Meyer (eds), *Understanding Care Homes: A Research and Development Perspective*, pp. 9–22. London: Jessica Kingsley Press.

Froggatt, K., Brazil, K., Hockley, J., and Reitinger, E. (2011) Improving Care for Older People Living and Dying in Long-Term Care Settings: A Whole System Approach. In: M. Gott, and C. Ingleton (eds), *Living with Ageing and Dying: Palliative and End of Life Care for Older People*, pp. 215–25. Oxford: Oxford University Press.

Heimerl, K. (2006) *Palliative Care in Organisationen umsetzen*. Wien: Habilitationsschrift.

Heimerl, K. (2008) *Orte zum Leben—Orte zum Sterben*. Palliative Care in Organisationen umsetzen. Freiburg: Lambertus.

Heintel, P. (2003) Interventionsforschung. In: E. Schmide (ed.), *Interventionswissenschaft—Interventionsforschung. Erörterung zu einer Prozesswissenschaft vor Ort, Band 2*, pp. 21–6. Klagenfurt: Klagenfurter Beiträge zur Interventionsforschung.

Heller, A., Dinges, S., Heimerl, K., Reitinger, E., and Wegleitner, K. (2003) Palliative Kultur in der stationären Altenhilfe. *Zeitschrift für Gerontologie und Geriatrie*, **36**(5): 360–65.

Heller, A., Heimerl, K., and Husebø, S. (eds) (2007) *Wenn nichts mehr zu machen ist, ist noch viel zu tun. Wie alte Menschen würdig sterben können*, 3rd edn. Freiburg: Lambertus.

Hochschild, A. (1983) *The Managed Heart: Commercialization of Human Feeling*. Berkeley, Los Angeles, London: University of California Press.

Hochschild, A. (1995) The Politics of Culture: Traditional, Cold Modern, and Warm Modern Ideals of Care. *Social Politics: International Studies in Gender, State and Society*, **2**(3): 331–46.

Hockley, J. (2002) Organizational Structures for Enhancing Standards of Palliative Care. In: J. Hockley, and D. Clark (eds), *Palliative Care for Older People in Care Homes*, pp. 165–81. Buckingham: Open University Press.

Hockley, J. (2006) The Development of High Quality End of Life Care for Older People in Nursing Homes: An Action Research Study. Unpublished PhD thesis: University of Edinburgh.

Hockley, J. and Clark, D. (2002) *Palliative Care for Older People in Care Homes*. Buckingham: Open University Press.

James, V. (2009) Positioning Emotion through the Body and Bodywork: A Reflection through Nursing as Craft. *International Journal of Work Organisation and Emotion*, **3**(2): 146–60.

Kojer, M. (2009) *Alt, krank und verwirrt. Einführung in die Praxis der Palliativen Geriatrie. 3. überarbeitete und erweiterte Auflage*. Freiburg im Breisgau: Lambertus.

Krainer, L. (2006) Interventionsforschung—eine Methode der Prozessethik? In: P. Heintel, L. Krainer, and M. Ukowitz (eds), *Beratung und Ethik. Praxis, Modelle, Dimensionen*, pp. 92–119. Berlin: Leutner.

Kreutzner, G. (2006) Care for Old People between Gender Relations, Gender Roles and Gender Constructs. In: G.M. Backes, V. Lasch, and K. Reimann (eds), *Gender, Health and Ageing: European Perspectives on Life Course, Health Issues and Social Challenges*, pp. 293–316. Wiesbaden: VS-Verlag.

Lamnek, S. (2005) *Qualitative Sozialforschung. Lehrbuch. 4. Auflage*. Weinheim: Beltz-PVU.

Lehner, E. and Reitinger, E. (2008) Gender-Analyse ethischer Entscheidungen in der Altenbetreuung. In: E. Reitinger (ed.), *Transdisziplinäre Praxis. Forschen im Sozial- und Gesundheitswesen*, pp. 137–52. Heidelberg: Systemische Forschung im Carl-Auer Verlag.

Pleschberger, S. (2007) Dignity and the Challenge of Dying in Nursing Homes: The Residents' View. *Age Ageing*, **(2)**: 197–202.

Reitinger, E. (2006) *Bedürfnismanagement in der stationären Altenhilfe. Systemtheoretische Analyse empirischer Evidenzen*. Heidelberg: Systemische Forschung im Carl-Auer Verlag.

Reitinger, E. (2008) *Transdisziplinäre Praxis. Forschen im Sozial-und Gesundheitswesen*. Heidelberg: Systemische Forschung im Carl-Auer Verlag.

Reitinger, E. and Heimerl, K. (2008) Ethische Entscheidungen im Alten-und Pflegeheim: Das Forschungsdesign. In: E. Reitinger (ed.), *Transdisziplinäre Praxis. Forschen im Sozial-und Gesundheitswesen*, pp. 89–108. Heidelberg: Systemische Forschung im Carl-Auer Verlag.

Reitinger, E. and Lehner E. (2009) Gender: Ethical Issues in Long Term Care. *European Journal of Palliative Care. Committed to People*. Abstracts. 11th Congress of the EAPC. Vienna 7–10 May 2009: 166.

Ribbens, J. and Edwards, R. (1998) *Feminist Dilemmas in Qualitative Research: Public Knowledge and Private Lives*. London: Sage.

Riley, S., Schouten, W., and Cahill, S. (2003) Exploring the Dynamics of Subjectivity and Power Between Researcher and Researched (62 paragraphs). *FQS-Forum Qualitative Social Research*, **4**(2) http://www.nbn-resolving.de/urn:nbn:de:0114-fqs0302400 (accessed: 26 July 2011).

Sandhu, H., Adams, A., Singleton, L., Clark-Carter, D., and Kidd, J. (2009) The Impact of Gender Dyads on Doctor-Patient Communication: A Systematic Review. *Patient Education and Counseling*, **76**(3): 348–55.

Schmitz, S. (2006) Geschlechtergrenzen. Geschlechtsentwicklung, Intersex und Transsex im Spannungsfeld zwischen biologischer Determination und kultureller Konstruktion. In: Ebelling, S. and Schmitz, S. (eds), *Geschlechterforschung und Naturwissenschaften. Einführung in ein komplexes Wechselspiel*, pp. 33–56. Wiesbaden: VS Verlag.

Small, N., Froggatt, K., and Downs, M. (2007) *Living and Dying with Dementia: Dialogues about Palliative Care*. Oxford: Oxford University Press.

Twigg, J. (2006) *The Body in Health and Social Care*. Hampshire: Palgrave Macmillan.

West, C. and Zimmerman, D.H. (1987) Doing Gender. *Gender & Society*, **2**(1): 125–51.

WHO (2003) *Gender, Health and Ageing: Gender and Health Information Sheet*. Geneva: WHO.

Yin, R. (1994) *Case Study Research: Design and Methods*, 3rd edn. Thousand Oaks: Sage.

Chapter 14

Demonstrating quality and rigour in action research: peer education for end-of-life issues

Katherine Froggatt

Introduction

Ensuring that high quality research is undertaken is an important issue that requires addressing whatever the study design is. This chapter considers the quality of action research, why it is important to address this issue, and offers some approaches that can be used to enable judgements about the quality of action research. Drawing upon an example of one study undertaken to develop and pilot a peer education programme on end-of-life issues for older people I illustrate how researchers can demonstrate the quality of their work.

Issues of quality

As in all research approaches there is a concern within action research to ensure that the highest quality research is undertaken. A discussion about how such judgments about quality are made is not unique to action research; such debates are also seen within positivist and interpretivist research paradigms.

A consideration of the quality of positivist research is conventionally addressed through attention being paid to issues of validity and reliability (Badger, 2000). This is based upon the premises of logical positivism and the existence of an objective reality. Within a qualitative paradigm quality has been framed in terms of different sets of concepts. See, for example, Guba and Lincoln's (1994) articulation of authenticity criteria:

- Fairness—concerned with the involvement of research participants in the process.
- Ontological authenticity—demonstration of evidence that participants have had their personal views changed.
- Educative authenticity—that participants understand better the views of others.
- Catalytic and tactical authenticity—that participants have been encouraged and empowered to change their culture on the basis of their new awareness.

As exemplified above, within qualitative research greater attention is paid to the under-pinning values that shape the research focus and process, the subjective role of the researcher and the rigour of the processes used within the research.

The relevance of the concepts of reliability and validity to participatory action research approaches can be questioned (Hope and Waterman, 2003). The criticism of action research from a positivist perspective is that the findings are site and context specific and therefore not necessarily generalizable. Two responses to this critique address the nature of truth and objectivity in research (Whitelaw *et al.*, 2003). Within a participatory paradigm, truth is not understood as a single objective thing but rather a multiple concept with its roots in power and values (McNiff, 2002). There is also recognition that the researcher is not seen as detached and objective; rather that engagement by the researcher with the participants and setting is inevitable.

Different ways forward to address the quality and rigour of action research have been described (Whitelaw *et al.*, 2003; Williamson *et al.*, 2012). It has been proposed that action researchers need to be more explicit about what they are doing (Marshall, 2001; McNiff, 2002; Reason, 2007) and demonstrate rigour in their use of methods. Alternatively, a relativist position (Mays and Pope, 2000) proposes that rather than follow the approach adopted within positivism or interpretivism a broader understanding of 'valid' is required (Reason and Bradbury, 2001). This is demonstrated by emphasis being placed upon the researcher and their values rather than the focus being upon methodology and its inherent rigour.

Williamson *et al.* (2012) have collated and reviewed a number of different approaches taken to assess the quality of action research. They identify five key issues present within the work of the authors reviewed:

- Generation of new knowledge
- Production of change
- Presence of an ethic of participation
- Demonstration of rigour in methods adopted
- Transferable and relevant to other contexts beyond the site of the study

(Williamson *et al.*, 2012: 223)

Williamson *et al.* acknowledge the challenge of undertaking this type of evaluation within action research, and the tension of fully representing complexity, whilst also offering a means to provide comparable information about the quality of studies.

Three broad tests of rigour for action research have been identified in the literature (Whitelaw *et al.*, 2003) concerned with principles, practicalities, and levels of process. These approaches are not necessarily mutually exclusive. Working with principles is concerned with demonstrating an adherence to a coherent set of principles within a participatory framework. Depending upon the principles identified as key for the approach taken (see Chapter 1), then what is required is a demonstration of how these have been used to shape the study through reflexivity and a dialectical critique. One way to do this is for the researcher to consciously pay attention to their beliefs and values through a high level of self-awareness, while at the same time seeking to represent the experience and evaluation of those participating in the research. This is done through reflexivity and the keeping of field notes as part of challenging the researcher in the light of differing opinions. In using a critical perspective the identification and subsequent exploration of tensions and contradictions within the researcher and the

Table 14.1 Development of ÄVS criteria from authenticity criteria

Authenticity criteria (adapted from: Guba and Lincoln, 1994)	ÄVS criteria (Nolan *et al.*, 2003)
Fairness	Equal access to all participants
Ontological authenticity	Enhanced awareness of self and situation
Educative authenticity	Enhanced awareness of others' situations
Catalytic authenticity	Encouraging action by identifying areas for change
Tactical authenticity	Enabling action by facilitating change

Nolan *et al.*, Gauging Quality in Constructivist Research: The Äldreväst Sjuhärad (ÄVS) model revisited, Quality in Ageing: *Policy, Practice and Research*, **4**(2): 22–7, copyright © 2003.

practice area can occur (Waterman, 1998). Using reflexivity to the fullest extent in exploring such issues can help demonstrate the transparency of an action research study (see Marshall, 2001, for examples of how this can be undertaken).

At least two frameworks have been developed that facilitate such a reflexive critique (Nolan *et al.*, 2003; Reason, 2007). The ÄVS model (Nolan *et al.*, 2003) has been used to make a judgement about the nature of participation within collaborative work with older people concerning end-of-life issues (Clarke *et al.*, 2009). This model draws upon the work of Guba and Lincoln (1994) and their authenticity criteria (Table 14.1). Work by Nolan *et al.* (2003) has adapted these principles for a participatory context and criteria relevant for this research paradigm: equality of access for participants; enhanced awareness by participants of themselves and their situation and also of other people's perspectives; the identification of areas for change; and the actual facilitation of change.

Reason (2007) has also developed quality criteria for action research based on the premise that action research contains many choices, and quality can be judged by looking at the way in which these choices are transparently identified and addressed with awareness. Four criteria are proposed that can be used to demonstrate the quality of action research with respect to its core values:

◆ The extent to which worthwhile practical purposes are addressed.

◆ The levels of democracy and participation in the processes of change.

◆ The different forms of knowledge engaged with during the study.

◆ The extent to which the research has been and continues to be responsive and developmental.

(Reason, 2007)

A consideration of the practicalities of action research methods is linked to the ability to demonstrate how the principles underpinning action research have been adhered to. This is a more pragmatic way of presenting the decision making and actual delivery of the action research study. A number of practical checklists exist (Titchen, 1999; Waterman *et al.*, 2001) that can be used to help demonstrate the quality of action research.

With respect to the levels of process, McNiff *et al.* (1996) propose a tripartite way to assess and understand quality that reflects the three levels of inquiry (Reason and Torbert, 2001): first person (internal), second person (external validation with others), and third person (wider public acknowledgement of the process and findings) (see Chapter 5). This approach is not incompatible with the principles and practical methods described above, and offers a way to structure such an evaluative process looking at how the research processes have been undertaken in different dimensions of the research.

Using the ÄVS model (Nolan *et al.*, 2003), I illustrate how this approach can be used to help consider the quality of participation within one action research study, developing public awareness of end-of-life issues for older adults. The background to the study and its design are described and I then use the ÄVS model to review how participative the study was for the participants.

Peer education for older adults about end-of-life issues

National end-of-life care strategies within England have indicated a need to raise the profile of end-of-life care and to change attitudes to death and dying in society (DH, 2008). With an ageing population, older adults increasingly need to address a number of life transitions (Hall *et al.*, 2011), such as where to live, where to be cared for, how to access resources, and where and how to attend to their last days of living. Improving older adults' awareness about end-of-life issues may help them to make informed choices and engage in timely end-of-life discussions with family and friends that will ultimately impact upon service provision. This action research study builds upon previous research undertaken to develop a peer education programme for end-of-life care education among older people (Seymour *et al.*, 2011). A group of eight older adults and one academic researcher from the North of England attended this programme. On the basis of this training the group undertook to develop community approaches to improving public awareness of end-of-life issues in their locality, using a participatory action research approach.

The study was undertaken with the aim to collaboratively develop end-of-life care planning resources and skills for raising public awareness of end-of-life issues for older people within one local setting (Froggatt *et al.*, 2010).

Methods

The research approach adopted for this study reflected the values of the group undertaking the work and the aims outlined above. The end-of-life peer education group comprised members of the public from the locality who were working with a researcher from a local university. All members were interested in and committed to improving public awareness of the issues older people faced as they look to the future and face end-of-life issues. The group collectively identified these areas for engagement with public awareness and end-of-life issues.

Action research places emphasis on collaborative working between multiple partners in gaining practical knowledge to effect change (Waterman *et al.*, 2001). Two key features of a participatory approach structured how the study was designed and undertaken: working with people, and the use of cycles of action and reflection. In this study the participants researched their own practice (first person inquiry) and also worked with others to raise awareness of end-of-life issues and bring about change (second person inquiry) (see Chapter 5).

Two strands of work were addressed: strand 1 focused upon the development of personal end-of-life information and resources portfolio; strand 2 focused upon the delivery of community workshops on end-of-life issues. In the study, ongoing cycles of action and reflection were followed, both individually and collectively. Each stage of action was followed by evaluation and then a period of reflection to feed into the next stage of action. Prospective and retrospective analysis was undertaken on the process and outcomes of the study using synthesis of thematic issues and template coding of evaluative elements (Crabtree and Miller, 1999).

The study was ethically reviewed and approved by an ethics committee at the host university. Attention was paid during the study to issues of consent, confidentiality, and potential distress for the project team and participants. In any discussion of issues around the end of life, bereavement, and loss there was the potential for emotional distress to be experienced by any of the participants (project team and workshop participants). In the workshops, provision was made to ensure that immediate support was available for individuals, should they require it, during or after the workshop. Written information was also provided about local sources of support for people requiring this following the events.

The two strands are presented consecutively, incorporating the methods and findings within each strand.

Strand 1: Development of personal end-of-life information and resources portfolio

Members of the peer education group first considered information needs regarding end-of-life issues, either for themselves or for family and friends close to them. A series of eight monthly meetings were held and end-of-life issues faced by group members were examined. Current resources available were identified and reviewed to ascertain the best elements of these resources, and note the weaknesses which could then be addressed. From this work, a personal portfolio within which individuals could record their information and resources pertinent to their issues was written and designed by the team. Notes were made of the discussions of each meeting and the decision making processes undertaken.

The process by which the personal portfolio was developed entailed the following elements of work. These processes were often undertaken concurrently and not always in the sequential way presented here.

Examination of end-of-life issues faced by group members

A wide range of issues were identified at the start of the project by the members of the core group concerned with communication issues and information needs prior to, during, and after death, and the services and resources available at these different times.

Identification of sources of information and resources to address these issues

The team sought to identify the resources available that would enable them to answer their own questions about these issues. Resources provided during the previous peer education training and further searches for information led to a collection of material that covered a wide range of issues that included advance care planning, mental capacity issues, powers of attorney, wills, and funerals. With the recognition that much information about planning already existed, it was agreed that the purpose of developing the portfolio was to create a holding document for the recording of personal information. Other sources of information and guidance would be signposted as required.

Review of resources and information

A number of key national resources were identified by the team as being of particular relevance to our work. These were collected and reviewed in terms of their purpose, content, strengths and weaknesses, and their contribution towards the development of our own portfolio.

Design and development of portfolio to record personal information

From the review of current material a number of issues about the nature of the content and design of the portfolio became clear. The contents of the portfolio needed to address:

- Biographical and personal details
- Health status and current care information
- Future planning for care

This led to the identification of eight sections within which the relevant information could be collated (Table 14.2).

Sharing the portfolio with workshop participants and further revision

Once the portfolio was agreed in a draft format it was used within the workshop to aid discussion about end-of-life issues. Each workshop participant was given a copy of the portfolio and asked to send their feedback back to the research team.

Using the portfolio

Throughout this work, members of the peer education group were also using the portfolio to support their personal thinking and planning. The portfolio has been used in a number of ways by members of the project team. Some have used it extensively to systematically document their personal information and wishes. Other have not been able to complete the documentation in the portfolio but used it to direct discussions with family members.

Strand 2: Development of a community workshop on end-of-life issues

Work was also undertaken to engage with older adults and their advocates (family members, paid care staff, and other health and social care professionals and volunteers

Table 14.2 Portfolio contents

Introduction to the portfolio

---

1. Who am I?

   An account of the person in words, pictures, audio recordings.

2. Personal details

   Information about the person and next of kin which someone could locate quickly in an emergency.

3. Life contacts

   Contact details of people significant to the individual.

4. Health information

   Information concerning health needs, medical, and care requirements.

5. Important documents

   List and details of where important documents/information are located.

6. How I want to be cared for now and in the future

   A person's preferences and wishes regarding care now and in the future.

7. Anticipating future changes

   Planning for a time when an individual might not be able to communicate his/her wishes and preferences within the current legal frameworks.

8. After I die

   Plans for funerals and other remembrance events after a person's death.

Further information

Resources

Background

---

who support and work with older adults). Two community end-of-life workshops were planned and delivered; the first workshop recruited older adults, the second primarily older people's advocates. The workshops were structured to address three specific areas:

1. What are some things to think about?
2. Starting to plan
3. Talking about these issues

The emphasis was upon an individual's engagement with these issues for his/herself, even if attending in a professional capacity. Attention was paid at the start of the workshop to issues of confidentiality, personal safety in that what people chose to disclose was their choice, the need to respect personal stories and not judge them, and also that support was available if required. An evaluation of the community workshops was undertaken using a post-workshop evaluation form distributed and collected on the day, and post-event reflections by members of the peer education group.

Thirty-five participants attended two community workshops. Twenty-one participants attended workshop 1 for older adults; 18 (81%) women and 3 (19%) men, and all 21 participants were over 55 years old. Workshop 2 which was aimed at the advocates of older people was attended by 14 participants, of whom one was an older adult. The other participants were health and social care workers based in hospital, hospice, care home, and voluntary sector settings working with older adults, palliative care, renal, and oncology patients in medical, social work, nursing, and other thera-peutic practices. Three men and eleven women participated.

Quality and rigour of this research

Drawing on the ÄVS model (Nolan *et al.*, 2003) I will show how in this study the peer education group were able to apply the principles to the processes adopted by the core peer educator group (Table 14.3). The data drawn on to support this discussion was derived from the peer education group meeting notes, post-event notes by the peer educators, and the post-workshop evaluation survey.

The principle of equal access was addressed for both the peer educators and work-shop participants. The core group of peer educators met monthly and worked together to shape the design of the portfolio and workshops. All the peer educators' views were heard during the core group meetings. The workshops were designed to facilitate dis-cussion in small groups around a table. This generally worked well, but one venue was less good for this type of discussion because of its size and was too noisy for people with hearing difficulties. In general, though, the ability to share experiences was val-ued, as can be demonstrated by a quote from the post-workshop written evaluation: 'Sharing of personal accounts. The facilitated table discussions were a good way of organizing it' (workshop 1 participant—older person). In terms of enhanced aware-ness about themselves and others it was clear that each member of the peer education

Table 14.3 Application of ÄVS principles

Principle	As applied in the study for the core peer educator group	As applied in the study for workshop participants
Equal access to all participants	Were the peer educators' views heard during the study?	Were workshop participants able to have their views heard?
Enhanced awareness of self and situation	Were the peer educators able to demonstrate enhanced awareness about end-of-life advance care planning and information giving?	Did workshop participants demonstrate enhanced awareness about end-of-life advance care planning and information giving?
Enhanced awareness of others' situations	Were the peer educators able to consider new ways of having discussions and sharing information as a consequence of being in the study?	Did workshop participants identify any actions they would undertake as a result of attending the workshop?
Encouraging action by identifying areas for change	Following the project were the peer educators able to share information and facilitate end-of-life discussions in their communities?	Was there any evidence that actions were undertaken by workshop participants?

Data Nolan *et al.*, Gauging quality in constructivist research: The Äldreväst Sjuhärad (ÄVS) model revisited, Quality in Ageing: Policy, Practice and Research, Issue 4, Volume 2, pp. 22–27, copyright © 2003.

group had a commitment to this work arising from personal and professional experiences. Therefore, each person was addressing particular issues of relevance to him or her. Initial meetings were focused upon hearing and understanding the different perspectives and experiences people brought to this work. It also allowed the peer element of education to be manifested in the group, as learning and knowledge was shared between members. Peer educators were also able to demonstrate enhanced awareness about end-of-life advance care planning and information given both within the core group meetings, and also as they engaged with the design and delivery of the two workshops. The workshops created a further space for personal learning of new information about end-of-life issues and also others' understandings of these issues. In the workshops, the initial focus on identifying the issues the participants were seeking to address indicated that they had come with many questions and a desire to find out more information and knowledge to help them answer their questions. The approach used in the workshops used personal stories to convey information about end-of-life issues and personal planning. This medium led to workshop participants identifying new understanding about these issues.

Action was encouraged and enabled in this study. A key aim for the project was to design a planning document and also to engage through workshops with other members of the general public. Therefore, the peer educators considered different ways of having discussions with other people and sharing information and then undertook this within the workshops, and also with their own families and friends: 'For me it has been important to complete the portfolio and take the necessary steps, which are important for me, at a time when I am not facing a major health crisis and therefore the hard work has been done and now can be put to rest until needed' (peer educator). It was more difficult to evaluate this aspect of the process for the workshop participants, as there was no follow-up after the workshops. However, there were indications on the post-workshop evaluation of actions individuals planned to do both with family members and for professionals with patients/clients: 'It has really spurred me on to talk to my parents about this' (workshop 2 participant— healthcare professional). This evaluative framework has allowed specific questions to be asked about the process of action research and to what extent it has been undertaken in a rigorous way.

Conclusion

Debates about the quality of action research address deeper questions of epistemology, as the concepts associated with quality (reliability, validity, rigour) are shaped by the paradigmatic origins of the research being undertaken. Within action research there is a recognition of the need to ensure that the research undertaken is of a high quality, and a number of different ways to undertake this have been proposed drawing on different frameworks (principle based, practical, typologies of level). Attention to these issues will enhance the quality of action research undertaken.

Acknowledgements

Thanks go to the peer educators for their enthusiasm and commitment to this project. Funding for the study described here was provided by NHS North Lancashire. I also acknowledge the work of Jane Seymour and Amanda Clarke which has helpfully informed what has been presented here.

References

Badger, T.G. (2000) Action Research: Change and Methodological Rigour. *Journal of Nursing Management*, **8**: 201–7.

Clarke, A., Sanders, C., Seymour, J.E., Gott, M., and Welton, M. (2009) Evaluating a Peer Education Programme for Advance End of Life Care Planning for Older Adults: The Peer Educators' Perspective. *International Journal of Disabilities and Human Development*, **8**, (1), 33–41.

Crabtree, B.F. and Miller, W.L. (1999) Using Codes and Code Manuals: A Template Organizing Style of Interpretation. In: B.F. Crabtree and W.L. Miller (eds), *Doing Qualitative Research*, 2nd edn, pp. 163–77. Newbury Park, California: Sage.

Department of Health (2008) End of Life Care Strategy—Promoting High Quality Care For All Adults at the End of Life. London: Department of Health.

Froggatt, K. with the Lancaster Peer Education Group: Capstick, C., Coles, O., Jacks, D., Lockett, S., McGill, I., Robinson, J., and Ross-Mills, J. (2010) *Improving Public Awareness of End of Life Issues among Older People in North Lancashire: A Peer Education Approach*. Final Report for NHS North Lancashire. Lancaster: Lancaster University.

Guba, E.G. and Lincoln, Y.S. (1994) Competing Paradigms in Qualitative Research. In: N.K. Denzin and Y.S. Lincoln (eds) *The Handbook of Qualitative Research*, pp. 105–17. Thousand Oaks, CA: Sage

Hall, S., Petkova, H., Tsouros, A.D., Costantini, M., and Higginson, I.J. (eds) (2011) *Palliative Care for Older People: Better Practices*. Copenghagen: WHO Regional Office for Europe.

Hope, K. and Waterman H. (2003) Praiseworthy Pragmatism? Validity and Action Research. *Journal of Advanced Nursing*, **44**(2), 120–27.

Lincoln, Y.S. and Guba, E.G. (2000) Paradigmatic Controversies, Contradictions and Emerging Confluences In: N.K. Denzin and Y.S. Lincoln (eds), *Handbook of Qualitative Research*, 2nd edn, pp. 163–88. Thousand Oaks, CA: Sage

Marshall, J. (2001) Self-Reflective Inquiry Practices. In: P. Reason and H. Bradbury (eds), *Handbook of Action Research. Participative Inquiry and Practice*. pp. 433–39. London: Sage.

Mays, N. and Pope, C. (2000) Qualitative Research in Health Care. Assessing Quality in Qualitative Research. *BMJ*, **320**: 50–52.

McNiff, J. (2002) *Action Research Principles and Practice*, 2nd edn. Abingdon: Routledge Falmer.

McNiff, J., Lomax, P., and Whitehead, J. (1996) *You and Your Action Research Project*. London: Routledge.

Nolan, M., Hanson, E., Magnusson, L., and Anderssonm, B.A. (2003) Gauging Quality in Constructivist Research: The Äldreväst Sjuhärad (ÄVS) model revisited. *Quality in Ageing—Policy, Practice and Research*, **4**(2): 22–7.

Reason, P. (2007) Choice and Quality in Action Research. *Journal of Management Inquiry*, **15**(2), 187–203.

Reason, P. and Bradbury, H. (2001) Inquiry and Participation in Search of a World Worthy of Human Aspiration. In: P. Reason and H. Bradbury (ed.), *Handbook of Action Research. Participative Inquiry and Practice*, pp. 1–14. London: Sage.

Reason, P. and Torbert, W.R. (2001) The Action Turn: Toward a Transformational Social Science. *Concepts and Transformations*, **6**(1), 1–37.

Seymour, J., Almack, K., Kennedy, S. and Froggatt, K. (2011) Peer Education for Advance Care Planning: Volunteers' Perspectives on a Training Programme and Community Engagement Activities, *Health Expectations*, doi: 10.1111/j.1369-7625.2011.00688.x.

Titchen, A. (1999) Issues of Validity in Action Research, *Nurse Researcher*, 2(3), 38–48.

Waterman, H. (1998) Embracing Ambiguities and Valuing Ourselves: Issues of Validity in Action Research. *Journal of Advanced Nursing*, **28**(1), 101–5.

Waterman, H., Tillen, D., Dickson, R., and de Koning, K. (2001) Action Research: A Systematic Review and Guidance for Assessment. *Health Technology Assessment*, **5**(23).

Whitelaw, S., Beattie, A., Balogh, R., and Watson, J. (2003) *A Review of the Nature of Action Research*. Cardiff: Welsh Assembly Government.

Williamson, G.R., Bellman, L., and Webster, J. (2012) *Action Research for Nursing and Healthcare*. London: Sage Publications.

Chapter 15

Addressing sustainability: a hospital-based action research study

Geralyn Hynes

Palliative care policy in many countries refers to the need for all healthcare professionals working in clinical care to have basic palliative care skills, while those working in specialist areas may advance to intermediate level palliative care practice. This means that palliative care principles should be practiced by all healthcare professionals. It is based on the assumption that many patients with progressive and advanced disease can have their care needs met comprehensively and satisfactorily, without referral to specialist palliative care units or personnel. Intermediate level palliative care refers to that which implies additional training and experience in palliative care among healthcare professionals who are not engaged full time in palliative care.

Establishing basic and intermediate level palliative approaches to care raises immediate questions about how palliative care becomes embedded in everyday practice across different care settings. In a busy medical ward within any acute hospital, where care is provided at a fast pace and the focus is on treatment of illness episodes as discrete events, embedding palliative care requires attention to and altering core values and assumptions that underpin existing practice. This reflects double loop learning as described by Argyris (2006). As already described (see Chapter 5), single loop learning occurs when a problem is addressed while holding to existing values, attitudes, and frameworks. However, double loop learning occurs when underlying values, attitudes, norms, and frameworks are tackled and modified. It is this double loop learning that enables sustainable change.

This chapter will explore the significance and challenges of sustaining an action research initiative. I will draw on the experiences of a project aimed at developing respiratory nursing practice within the acute hospital context to address palliative care in advanced chronic obstructive pulmonary disease (COPD) to highlight issues of sustainability in action research. There is a significant emphasis within the action research community on issues of sustainability from an ecological and environmental perspective. However, I use the term to reflect its older use: capacity to be continued or bear up.

I begin with the importance of confronting existing values and assumptions of practice as key to long-term sustainability. Following that, I describe the project, with particular emphasis on the challenge of sustaining an inquiry process in a way that fosters long-term questioning of practice and movement towards embedding palliative care in everyday practice. In the final section, I draw on the idea of an 'attitude of inquiry' as being central to sustainability in action research.

Confronting existing values and assumptions about practice

Challenges of embedding basic palliative care in practice

Palliative care policy in Ireland and the UK is unequivocal in terms of the need to embed palliative care in everyday practice across different care settings, specialisms, and disciplines. Difficulties persist in embedding palliative care across different health-care systems (Gott *et al.*, 2001; 2012). Reasons for this may reflect interventions that address 'single' rather than 'double loop' learning in settings where the core assumptions, values, attitudes, and frameworks for practice are not addressed. Typically, in an acute medical care environment into which patients experiencing exacerbations of advanced chronic illnesses such as COPD are admitted, care delivery is focused on the exacerbation as a discrete episode and managed accordingly. Those patients deemed to have palliative care needs may be referred to the specialist palliative care teams for symptom management, resulting in concerns about reducing palliative care to a series of competencies or technical control of symptoms (RCP London, 2007).

The philosophy of palliative care is underpinned by the notion of total pain in advanced illness (Richmond, 2005). Total pain recognizes that pain is multidimensional with physical, psycho-social, emotional, and existential dimensions. These are interdependent; to focus on one dimension only, such as physical pain, is to deny understanding of a person's total pain or suffering. In advanced COPD, for instance, patients' illness accounts refer to living a life of COPD in which exacerbations are seen in terms of the overall illness trajectory (Elkington *et al.*, 2004; Fraser *et al.*, 2006; Goodridge, 2006; Goodridge *et al.*, 2008). Thus, care delivery that focuses on management of exacerbations as discrete episodes fails to acknowledge patients' total pain or suffering and therefore palliative care needs.

Engaging with different care philosophies

To embed palliative care at basic and intermediate level into an acute care environment requires a change in thinking or different model reflecting double loop learning (Argyris, 2006). For Argyris (2006), single loop learning is 'the detection and correction of errors that does not require changing the values that govern existing theory in use' (p. 10). Single loop learning occurs when a problem is identified and corrected in a way that permits the organization to carry on its present policies or achieve its present objectives. In contrast, double loop learning questions the status quo.

Embedding palliative care in everyday practice is not about supplanting one care approach with another. In the hospital environment, different world-views are expressed through articulation of care needs and approaches, assessments of care process, and organization of care. Attention to a patient's suffering experience reflects a different understanding of care needs to one which focuses on biomedical parameters, often referred to as disease-oriented care. The point here is not to denigrate any one approach to care. Rather, it is to draw attention to the complex interaction of all and often competing world-views that underpin approaches to care on a moment-to-moment basis. Put simply, a patient whose immediate problem is inability to breathe needs the healthcare professional to address the relevant biomedical markers and interventions as appropriate. Conversely, a patient who is facing increased disability and dependency requires an appreciation of the concept of total pain. Thus, embedding palliative care in everyday practice requires a moment-to-moment engagement with different understandings of the world through engaging with conflicting care philosophies.

Orders of change

Coghlan and Rashford (2006) describe first, second, and third order change. In first order change, a specific change is identified without any shift in existing ways of thinking. In second order change there is a shift in core assumptions, while third order change involves confronting fundamental and complex attitudinal and cultural issues towards questioning and changing assumptions about everyday practice. For an action research initiative to achieve such a third order change, the inquiry process needs to foster and sustain a shifting of core assumptions about acute care.

Second order change, while resulting in a modification of core assumptions, will over time take on a first order identity. It does not guarantee sustained change since the focus may be on the change rather than generating a process of continual questioning. Changes arising from some modification of basic assumptions may become entrenched and ritualized. Thus, practitioners need to develop a habit of continually questioning core assumptions about everyday practice, a habit which underscores third order change. This brings the focus to the inquiry process as one that nurtures questioning of core assumptions about practice. The focus of inquiry becomes questioning assumptions or one's own individual and professional world-view.

How then, does one create a space in an action research project that enables participants or co-researchers to tackle core assumptions about their everyday practice? How does an inquiry process seek to reconcile different and perhaps conflicting care philosophies in an environment in which different forms of evidence and voices of disciplines and patients are hierarchical? Action research recognizes the importance of participation as extending well beyond who sits around the table. Rather, participation is about engaging with *other*—where *other* may be person, culture, place, disciplinary world-view, or ways of understanding the world through different kinds of knowledge, etc. This view of participation invites an engagement with different care philosophies as a process of recognizing and being open to that which is *other*.

Principle of participation in action research

Participation in action research is informed by the idea of co-researching or researching 'with' rather than 'on' people (Reason and Bradbury, 2008). Participation has been described as being both epistemological and political (Reason, 2006; Reason and Bradbury, 2008). In the epistemological sense, researching with others means that inquiry is based on participants' understanding of the unfolding process and joint meaning-making rather than through the lens of a lead researcher's individual world-view. Participation requires full engagement, with plurality of knowing at both individual and group levels. Action research recognizes the ability and right of individuals to have a say in how knowledge is generated about them and the decisions that might affect them. In this sense, participation is political (Gaventa and Cornwall, 2008; Kemmis, 2008), whether this is reflected in overt oppression or covert silencing through failure to recognize different world-views. In short, participation in action research recognizes meaning making in everyday practice as an intensely political affair.

First, second, and third person inquiry is integral to how we address participation in action research, as already described in Chapter 5. In other words, first person inquiry seeks to render conscious the choices made in moment-to-moment attention to voice or world-view, whether or not this is articulated to others. Second person inquiry draws attention to how individuals work with each other in the spirit of co-inquiry and joint meaning making (Coghlan and Brannick, 2010; Reason and Bradbury, 2008). At issue here is how people are part of an action research inquiry, who is involved, and the nature of the dialogic process of engagement. Issues, such as consensus, collusion, tensions in facilitation, and first order democracy (Reason, 2006), are tackled though attention to openness to and engagement with *other*. Third person inquiry is addressed through meetings and dissemination of results, publishing or extending the scope of action through a network (Gustavsen *et al.*, 2008).

Participation as engagement with *other* through first and second person inquiry underpins the idea of third order change. Engagement with *other* provided a framework for an action research project, to which I now turn.

Developing respiratory nursing practice to address the palliative care needs of patients with advanced COPD

Background

This project was based in an acute general hospital context and sought to develop respiratory nursing practice to address the palliative care needs of patients with advanced COPD (Hynes, 2010). Patients with advanced COPD live with severe breathlessness and experience life- threatening acute exacerbations requiring emergency hospital admissions. Palliative care for this patient group is made complex by a number of factors:

- Difficulties in assessing prognosis
- Complex treatment interventions that may be aggressive to the end
- The acute medical care environment as one that is more geared towards, if not cure, then management of 'an illness episode' and discharge

These factors can militate against conversations about death and dying, and involvement of the palliative care team. Increasingly, frequent admissions can obscure a 'standing back' to see an overall decline or the total pain of a patient. The advanced COPD trajectory reflects that of other advanced chronic illnesses seen in acute hospitals (Gott *et al.*, 2007; Health Service Executive and Irish Hospice Foundation, 2008; Lynn and Adamson, 2003).

The idea for this project emerged from a growing awareness among those of us involved in respiratory care. I had a background in respiratory nursing before moving into respiratory nursing education. I was also an active member of the respiratory nurses' association in Ireland. In the classroom and through the association, concerns were increasingly being raised about unmet palliative care needs of patients with advanced COPD. A respiratory nurse specialist from the hospital where this project took place had a particular interest in developing practice to address the palliative care needs of her patients. This led to the idea of an action research project. Thus, I was an outsider in the context of my relationship with the hospital. However, Herr and Anderson (2005) offer a more nuanced notion of insider/outsider roles. For example, my respiratory nursing background offered an insider status from the perspective of respiratory care.

The project was designed in collaboration with the two respiratory nurse specialists in the hospital and had two phases (see Figure 15.1). The first phase aimed to identify the palliative care needs of 26 patients through individual interviews. The findings illustrated high symptom burden, poor quality of life, and the interplay between living with severe breathlessness and suffering. Phase 1 provided a foundation for understanding patients' illness experiences. Phase 2 was a cooperative inquiry as a form of action research involving respiratory and palliative care nurses, and a nurse researcher (author). The intended outcome for this phase was to provide a framework for addressing and embedding palliative care in everyday advanced COPD care and is my focus here.

Cooperative inquiry is one in which 'all participants work together in an inquiry group as co-researchers and co-subjects' (Reason and Heron, 2008: 366). An inquiry

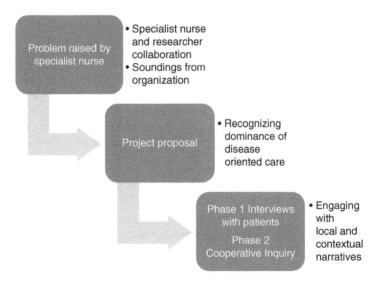

Fig. 15.1 Project roll-out.

group usually comes together to address a shared concern or interest. The group engages in cycles of action and reflection in a systematic approach to developing understanding and action. The aim of our cooperative inquiry was to make sense of respiratory nursing practice and explore how care needs identified in phase 1 might be addressed. Our inquiry into what palliative nursing care might mean in COPD rested on bringing together those nurses with palliative and respiratory care knowledge.

The cooperative inquiry (CI)

The cooperative inquiry (CI) group met over a 17-month period and was comprised of: respiratory and palliative care clinical nurse specialists; ward based clinical nurse managers; and me as an action researcher. I made notes from each CI meeting and circulated these in advance of the next meeting. We re-visited themes from the previous meeting at the start of each meeting. At 10, 16, and 17 months, the group reviewed the emerging themes. This process of agreeing and revisiting themes was intended to support a 'second order change' by focusing on participation in terms of both co-generation of practice-based knowledge and examining our engagement with the respective voices of palliative and acute medical care. By learning to challenge our different standpoints, namely: ward-based; specialist respiratory; and palliative care, I hoped to nurture the inquiry towards third order change.

Sustaining the inquiry process: working within practice constraints

Opening a space

The challenges of opening a space that respects dominant practices or ideas, or wish for quick action while also seeking to foster a 'standing back from these', have been articulated by others (Ospina *et al.*, 2004; Wicks and Reason, 2009). For our purposes here, I will focus on the initial steps in the inquiry process, sustaining the inquiry process, and ultimately engaging with the conflicts inherent with mediating both palliative and acute medical approaches to care in everyday practice.

Initially, and at the request of members, the time for meetings was limited to 30 minutes. However, this rule was relaxed by the third meeting and thereafter we checked at the start of each meeting what time pressures we were under and worked from that basis. In addition, there were informal meetings, often over lunch, that ranged from 30 minutes to over an hour. The 30-minute rule reflected the norm for clinical meetings and the difficulties members had at the outset in viewing the inquiry as something different. This was further illustrated in responses to my tentative questioning about what we needed to consider in relation to addressing palliative care in COPD. Discussion centred on the need for guidelines and protocols for the use of non-invasive ventilation and other clinical interventions at end of life; these were directed at the medical team in general, rather than nursing specifically.

At the same time, I invited the group to air concerns about the inquiry process. We identified three difficulties over the course of the first two meetings. First, we acknowledged our committee fatigue and wariness of additional workload that might spring from the project. Committees tend to generate work, especially for members, while also failing to address underlying problems pertaining to organizational politics or hierarchical teams and hegemony, that is, failing to achieve second and third order change. Second, we acknowledged our fears about engaging with patients' suffering and not being able to 'fix' or treat their distress. We were concerned about delving into what might seem insurmountable problems in terms of patients' psychosocial needs. Third, we were unsure about how much we could achieve within the clinical environment, and the hierarchical, resource, and organizational constraints therein.

I was acutely aware throughout the early meetings that the project was identified as Geralyn's research which had management support and so might be construed as requiring input but no ownership. In other words, my invitations to join the CI group may have resembled the more typical establishment of a work-based committee. As Wicks and Reason (2009) note, the initiating cooperative inquiry researcher proposes a topic, invites co-researchers to join and then introduces them to the inquiry, 'thus in formality and explicitness mimicking aspects of the system' (p. 247). By way of separating our inquiry from a more traditional view of inquiry or work-based committees, my intention was to make clear the principles of co-inquiring. At issue here is the perceived nature of collaboration initially and its impact on the quality of participation and choices made throughout the inquiry process. Using Cornwall's (1996) typology, it seemed important to move from the risk of perceived co-option being viewed as an outsider with management support and a pre-determined inquiry process. Cornwall sees this form of co-option akin to research 'on' rather than 'with' others. In contrast, co-learning or collective action points to reciprocity in the inquiry reflecting research by participants (Cornwall, 1996).

I was conscious of the difficulties for anyone coming to action research for the first time in an environment where practice-based meetings are normally driven by a tightly controlled agenda that is more often focused on policy and protocol matters. Among my first priorities was to find ways of enhancing reciprocity and freedom to develop our own understanding of respiratory nursing in advanced COPD. My initial positionality intersected with control, action, and voice (Ospina *et al.*, 2008). Ensuring the group had control over meeting arrangements was an early and easy step in responding to issues of control over the process. In consciously attending to the need to give ownership to the group and to place trust in the process as an emergent one, I voiced no reaction to the 30-minute limit imposed on the meetings. Later, as the process unfolded, the meetings gradually lengthened to over an hour and on occasion to nearly two hours. Less simple, however, was finding a balance between the need for laying a foundation towards finding our feet in the CI process, and responding to early calls for action.

Just as Arieli *et al.* (2009) struggled through layered and deeply rooted misunderstandings in their efforts to address participation, I found myself struggling between letting go my participatory ideals and, instead, attending fully to the early issues raised in the group. I was conscious that the early suggestions were rooted in traditional divisions between nursing and medicine, and the demands on practice versus those on management. When the need for guidelines and protocols was aired initially, I struggled against and often failed in being overly directive through talking about the theory of participation in action research and third order change. In acknowledging our concerns about the inquiry process and our past experiences of clinical meetings, we were at least pausing in that space between stimulus and response where the stimulus was coming together in a meeting forum and the response was our general misgivings and conditioning concerning how meetings are organized and their functions.

Engagement with other: working towards third order change

The CI findings illustrated two contradictory facets of respiratory nursing practice. In the first, respiratory care was disease oriented and underpinned by organizational dictates of what constitutes 'normal' care in terms of bed management, admission, and discharge procedures; appropriate time per patient consultation in the outpatients' department; and documentation procedures. Criteria for admission and discharge from hospital, and patient assessment in outpatients reflected a focus on a patient's oxygenation levels and related equipment and measurement. Similarly, levels of infection and other patho-physiological markers were a basis for disease-oriented care. Also, the hospital was constantly under pressure to provide beds for patients in need of hospital admission and manage waiting times for those who required outpatient care. Patients were often discharged home with little notice and limited support because of bed shortages. Criteria to discharge were based on patho-physiological markers with limited reference to illness-oriented needs. For the respiratory nurses and other team members, care was provided at a fast pace with limited scope for engagement with patients' illness-oriented concerns or experiences. Not surprisingly, there were difficulties in responding to patients' fears or needs for conversations about death and dying. The initial focus of the cooperative inquiry meetings was in line with disease-oriented care, risk management, and an emphasis on standardization of work procedures and practices.

In sharp contrast, the second facet of respiratory nursing was the close relationships built up with patients as their condition deteriorated and their hospital admissions increased in frequency. Shortly before the third CI group meeting, a patient died. Discussion centred on her death, events leading up to it, and a sense of loss. Questions opened up about failure or reluctance to have death and dying conversations with patients and relatives. 'Families, do you know if they could bring up the issues also because they run as far from it all the time, as we do, so I think it's like between all of us, like the patient, family and staff, we all run away' (Cooperative Inquiry Group Meeting, Hynes, 2010). The issue of concern for the group was that there had not occurred with her a conversation about death and dying. Members recalled instances when the patient had indirectly and in vain invited such conversations. The focus of the cooperative inquiry group shifted towards making sense of respiratory nursing practice in acute care, which members saw as at odds with their relationships with patients. 'You'd notice in OPD [outpatient department], like, if you give the time or you make the effort for time they will remember . . . whereas if it doesn't go well, you know, you rush someone, you get the feeling the next time that you didn't really give them enough time, you know. They do let you know' (Cooperative Inquiry Group Meeting, Hynes, 2010). In between admissions patients attended respiratory clinics and were supported by the respiratory clinical nurse specialists. The nurse/patient relationships built up over time gave rise to knowledge of individual patients' illness experiences. This illness awareness represented background knowledge or knowing the person as distinct from knowing the patient or case (Liaschenko, 1997). However, this knowing the patient or illness knowledge developed from informal or ad hoc conversations with patients. It was knowledge that stood outside formal engagement with patients, documentation, ward rounds, and multi-disciplinary team meetings.

Re/presentation of patients

Acknowledging a disease/illness dichotomy in our relationship with patients drew attention to different ways we re/presented patients in everyday practice. In our documentation and clinical conversations, we addressed biomedical markers and were reductionist or disease oriented in our talk. Typically, patients' needs were described in terms of symptom control and treatment self-efficacy. This was at odds with our illness knowledge of a patient derived from conversations about life events, struggles to maintain everyday routines with increasing disability and loss. Conversations such as these illustrated suffering. Attending to these conflicting re/presentations drew attention to our engagement with conflicting philosophies of care while privileging that of acute care.

Though we increasingly saw the centrality of 'knowing the person' to addressing palliative care needs, this was also knowledge that was not articulated in formalized accounts such as patient documentation and ward rounds. The idea of re/presentation highlighted the need to articulate and act on illness-oriented knowledge of patients' experiences and meaning making. In the acute care environment, attempting to privilege illness-oriented knowledge was an attempt to re-describe our understanding of care and the practice environment. In seeking to privilege illness-oriented knowledge, the respiratory nurses were engaging with the notion of suffering and attempts to embed palliative care within acute care.

However, engaging with suffering highlighted the gap between our idealized nursing care and the moral experience of living with compromises in the harsh reality of care delivery in the current Irish healthcare environment. Our idealized nursing care gave way to care practices driven by pressures of staffing levels, time pressures, ward routines, bed shortages, the need to discharge patients quickly with little notice, etc. Examples were aired of being aware of patients' wishes to speak about their fears but failing to meet this wish or diverting conversations towards safer territory. These examples illustrated the divided world and self in everyday practice. On the one hand, we could explain our inability to sit with distressed patients as evidence of system limitations; on the other hand, in acknowledging our close relationships with patients and our understanding of their illness experiences, we were faced with the duality of our responsibility to responding to their suffering and the requirements of the hospital system.

Actions and choice points: moving towards second order change

Our cooperative inquiry group drew back from our initial meetings and focus on guideline development. We entered into a space that sought to engage with conflicting philosophies and responses to care needs. Our inquiry period lacked overt confrontations with what we saw as system-wide dominant disease-oriented care. Rather, our actions fell into two categories. In the first, there was a shift in the inner self, perhaps best expressed in terms of stepping into dual citizenship. In the second category, small ad hoc actions reflected changes in practice, but together they were aimed at increasing awareness of palliative COPD care.

Actions as inner shifts

There was learning to acknowledge and respond to illness experiences as palliative COPD care. This meant accepting 'knowing the patient as person' as a legitimate type of healthcare knowledge and thus questioning our individual re/presentation of and responsibility to *other*. Examples of shifts in our thinking included confronting the significance of illness meaning making in patients' accounts. In one meeting, a respiratory nurse explored the significance for a patient of the loss of a pet that represented a link to the past. The pet and the past were bound together in the losses this patient had endured in her life history and was now experiencing in terms of her worsening condition. The nurse's subsequent difficulty in presenting this within the more typical format of patient documentation illustrated the gap between the patient's illness meaning making and system-wide re/presentation: 'Yeah you'd be thinking how can I put this down in a medical way?' (Cooperative Inquiry Group Meeting, Hynes, 2010). For the patient, the loss of her pet took on a huge significance in her current COPD state and suffering. Current symptoms were bound up in her sense of loss. However, for the nurse, by just focusing on current symptoms and self-management in the documentation, the significance of the pet and therefore the patient's suffering was erased. In this sense, the patient's symptoms and illness experience was *misrepresented* in the documentation.

Actions as confronting culture

Nurses sought to increase awareness of palliative care needs against a wider culture of limited engagement with the palliative care team. The respiratory nurses increasingly sought advice from the palliative care team and made a point of recording this advice in patient documentation in order to increase awareness of palliative care needs. Though the palliative care team could visit a patient only after the formal referral procedures were instigated, by giving 'advice' directly to the respiratory nurses, the cooperative inquiry group members were attempting to increase the visibility of palliative care while also supporting nurses to address care needs.

Small actions such as these might be better described as simply opening a conversation about palliative COPD as illness-oriented care. In these actions, the group members were inviting management and medicine to engage with a care philosophy that ran counter to the dominant acute care narratives. Such invitations were subtle rather than openly confrontational and were underpinned by an acknowledgement of multiple understandings of care needs.

In the end, sustainability for this project, if understood as embedding basic palliative care in everyday practice, was less about high profile protocols and interventions, but rather a process of becoming practiced at responding to our re/presentation of care needs on a moment-to-moment basis. In other words, sustainability was about embedding in our individual practice a questioning attitude towards our dual responsibility to the system and illness experiences of individual patients.

Nurturing sustainability: moving towards third order change

For Marshall and Reason (2007) an ongoing dialogue with the world and self underscores their idea of quality in research through taking an attitude of inquiry: 'This is a project with an ever-receding horizon rather than a state that can easily be achieved. Being willing to explore purposes, and being open to renewed insights into these, however provisional and shifting, is an underlying value in much of action research' (Marshall and Reason, 2007: 371). A feature of this notion of attitude of inquiry is that it is implicitly an open-ended process since it is, by definition, always open to question. Put simply, the action researcher in adopting an attitude of inquiry attends to increasing awareness of his/her frames of reference or horizon, engages with *other*, and remains open to contradictions and paradoxes rather than finalizing a state of play. Inquiry is therefore participative, always emerging and open to different world-views. The promise of sustainability rests on developing from the inquiry a habit of openness or an attitude of inquiry.

While I struggled to identify tangible outcomes that could be presented to management as evidence of addressing palliative care needs of patients with COPD, the inquiry had shifted towards a reflective process with what might be seen as limited action. Though more patients were being referred to the palliative care team, this was still ad hoc, and decision making was not linked to any framework for needs assessment. Typically, acknowledging first, the notion of suffering and second, the interconnection of bio-psychosocial emotional and existential pain, resulted in nurses seeking palliative care support. They still did not have confidence in their own ability to engage with their patients' experiences of suffering or total pain despite this reflecting basic level (level one) palliative care (Gott *et al.*, 2012). As a consequence, the palliative care clinical nurse specialist was now engaged in what could be construed as basic level palliative COPD care as nurses struggled with their engagement with patients' illness experiences.

The other group members strongly disagreed with my concerns and viewed as significant our formation as a cross palliative and respiratory care group, and our bringing to the fore our local moral world of nursing and struggles therein. For them, this was the base upon which to integrate palliative care into their COPD nursing care. They believed that a palliative care conscientization process was established in respect of their own individual practice and relayed examples of this from their interactions with patients and doctors. In essence, the inquiry as a process of opening and maintaining a conversation about palliative COPD care was of itself a framework, if an unconventional one, for developing respiratory nursing practice to address palliative care needs of patients with advanced COPD.

Conclusion

Organizations supporting action research may understandably look for clear changes in practice as the primary outcome, with possibly less emphasis on whether a change is of a first or second order nature. This can present a dilemma for the action researcher striving towards a third order change that reflects the development of a more habitual questioning of the values and assumptions underpinning practice. This might be understood as adopting an attitude of inquiry towards one's engagement with practice. However, promoting an attitude of inquiry within a new action research project is particularly challenged by the paradoxes concerning opening a space for inquiry in the spirit of co-inquiry with those entering an action research inquiry for the first time. Participants may lean toward single loop learning and first order change through a focus on guideline development, while the lead action researcher may have a double loop learning or third order change agenda. Addressing sustainability is thus, a complex and nuanced process that privileges the notion of an attitude of inquiry that is directed at and nurtured within the inquiry process itself from the outset.

References

Argyris, C. (2006) *Reasons and Rationalizations: The Limits to Organizational Knowledge.* Oxford: Oxford University Press.

Arieli, D., Friedman, V.J., and Agbaria, K. (2009) The paradox of Participation in Action Research. *Action Research*, 7: 263–90.

Coghlan, D. and Brannick, T. (2010) *Doing Action Research in Your Own Organization*, 3rd edn. London: Sage.

Coghlan, D. and Rashford, N.S. (2006) *Organizational Change and Strategy: An Interlevel Dynamics Approach.* Oxford: Routledge.

Cornwall, A. (1996) Towards Participatory Practice: Participatory Rural Appraisal (PRA) and the Participatory Process. In: K. De Koning and M. Martin (eds), *Participatory Research in Health: Issues and Experiences*, pp. 94–107. NPPHCN, London: Zed Books.

Elkington, H., White, P., Addington-Hall, J., Higgs, R., and Pettinari, C. (2004) The Last Year of Life of COPD: A Qualitative Study of Symptoms and Services. *Respiratory Medicine*, **98**: 439–45.

Fraser, D.D., Kee, C.C., and Minick, P. (2006) Living with Chronic Obstructive Pulmonary Disease: Insiders' Perspectives. *Journal of Advanced Nursing*, **55**: 550–58.

Gaventa, J. and Cornwall, A. (2008) Power and Knowledge. In: P. Reason and H. Bradbury (eds), *The Handbook of Action Research*, pp. 172–89. London: Sage.

Goodridge, D. (2006) People with Chronic Obstructive Pulmonary Disease at the End of Life: A Review of the Literature. *International Journal of Palliative Nursing*, **12**: 390–96.

Goodridge, D., Lawson, J., Duggleby, W., Marciniuk, D., Rennie, D., and Stang, M. (2008) Health Care Utilization of Patients with Chronic Obstructive Pulmonary Disease and Lung Cancer in the Last 12 Months of Life. *Respiratory Medicine*, **102**: 885–91.

Gott, C.M., Ahmedzai, S.H., and Wood, C. (2001) How Many Inpatients at an Acute Hospital Have Palliative Care Needs? Comparing the Perspectives of Medical and Nursing Staff. *Palliative Medicine*, **15**: 451–60.

Gott, M., Barnes, S., Parker, C., et al. (2007) Dying Trajectories in Heart Failure. *Palliative Medicine*, **21**: 95–9.

Gott, M., Seymour, J., Ingleton, C., Gardiner, C., and Bellamy, G. (2012) 'That's Part of Everybody's Job': The Perspectives of Health Care Staff in England and New Zealand on the Meaning and Remit of Palliative Care. *Palliative Medicine*, **26**(3): 232–41.

Gustavsen, B., Hansson, A., and Qvale, T.U. (2008) Action Research and the Challenge of Scope. In: P. Reason and H. Bradbury (eds), *The Handbook of Action Research*, 2nd edn, pp. 63–76. London: Sage.

Health Service Executive & Irish Hospice Foundation (2008) *Palliative Care for All: Integrating Palliative Care into Disease Management Frameworks*. Dublin: Irish Hospice Foundation.

Herr, K. and Anderson, G. (2005) *The Action Research Dissertation*. California: Sage.

Hynes, G. (2010) Dying to Breathe: A Conversation at the Crossroads of Respiratory and Palliative Nursing Care—An Action Research Project. Unpublished thesis: Trinity College, University of Dublin.

Kemmis, S. (2008) Critical Theory and Participatory Action Research. In: P. Reason and H. Bradbury (eds), *The Handbook of Action Research*, 2nd edn, pp. 121–38. London: Sage.

Liaschenko, J. (1997) Knowing the Patient In: S.E. Thorn and V.E. Hays (eds), *Nursing Praxis: Knowledge and Action*, pp. 23–38. Thousand Oaks: Sage.

Lynn, J. and Adamson, D.M. (2003) *Living Well at the End of Life: Adapting Health Care to Serious Chronic Illness in Old Age*. California: Rand Health.

Marshall, J. and Reason, P. (2007) Quality in research as 'Taking an Attitude of Inquiry' *Management Research News*, **30**(5): 368–80.

Ospina, S., Dodge, J., Godsoe, B. Minieri, J., Reza, S., and Schall, E. (2004) From Consent to Mutual Inquiry: Balancing Democracy and Authority in Action Research. *Action Research*, **2**: 47–69.

Ospina, S., Dodge, J., Foldy, E.G., and Hofmann-Pinilla, A. (2008) Taking the Action Turn: Lessons from Bringing Participation to Qualitative Research. In: P. Reason and H. Bradbury (eds), *The Handbook of Action Research*, 2nd edn, pp. 420–34. London: Sage.

Reason, P. (2006) Choice and Quality in Action Research Practice. *Journal of Management Inquiry,* **15**: 187–203.

Reason, P. and Bradbury, H. (2008) Introduction In: P. Reason and H. Bradbury (eds), *The Handbook of Action Research*, 2nd edn, pp. 1–10. London: Sage.

Reason, P. and Heron, J. (2008) Extending Epistemology within a Co-operative Inquiry. In: P. Reason and H. Bradbury (eds), *The Handbook of Action Research*, 2nd edn, pp. 366–80. London: Sage.

Richmond, C. (2005) Dame Cicely Saunders. *British Medical Journal*, **331**: 238.

Royal College of Physicians (2007) *Palliative Care Services: Meeting the Needs of Patients— Report of a Working Party*. London: Royal College of Physicians.

Wicks, P.G. and Reason, P. (2009) Initiating Action Research: Challenges and Paradoxes of Opening Communicative Space. *Action Research*, **7**: 243–62.

Chapter 16

Challenges for collaboration

Katherine Froggatt, Katharina Heimerl,
and Jo Hockley

Introduction

Participatory research and palliative care as research and practice disciplines, respectively, are both relatively young and increasing in prominence. These movements have arisen as a response to identified shortcomings and critique of the more dominant approaches to research and care provision for dying people. There is a further congruence between palliative care and participatory research in terms of holism. There is the holistic dynamic present within palliative care that seeks to address all of an individual's needs (physical, psychological, social, and spiritual), recognizing that the individual is located in a wider social network of family and friends (Sepulveda *et al.*, 2002). So too, research based on a participatory paradigm seeks to engage with the whole person in their whole context (Heimerl *et al.*, 2012; Hughes, 2008).

This chapter concludes this edited book by bringing together some key themes that have arisen through the accounts presented here in terms of the strengths, weaknesses, and existing gaps in the field. We use Ferlie and Shortell's (2001) typology of multiple levels of change to make some observations about the foci of participatory research in palliative care: at the individual, team, organizational, and the wider system level (Ferlie and Shortell, 2001). This perspective is strongly related to the 'levels to construct a system' as described in German systems theory (Willke, 2005) (see Chapter 3).

In undertaking participatory research in palliative care we encounter challenges that arise due to the fact that the research is participatory (challenges in *action* research), while other challenges originate in the field of palliative care (challenges of *palliative care* research). Some, maybe even most, challenges are situated at the intersection of both. The challenges of undertaking both participatory research and palliative care research have been well documented, and key aspects are considered here. We avoid the provision of easy answers to these challenges, but rather conclude with some key principles that may assist researchers and practitioners as they consider the relevance of this approach to their own practice and concerns.

Key threads

Within this book a number of current, or recently completed participatory action research projects have been presented. These studies are not exhaustive of participatory research that has been or is being undertaken within the palliative care field.

We are aware of a number of gaps that exist within this text with respect to the populations involved. Whilst there has been participatory research undertaken with children (Chowns, 2008), this is not represented here. Although specialist palliative care settings/hospices are included in some studies (White and Lynch, Chapter 9) they do not constitute the main focus in any of the chapters of the book. The majority of the studies included here address general care settings such as nursing homes, hospitals, and/or care in people's domestic homes. Research from countries outside the high income countries is also limited, although we are aware of innovative participatory research in India (Kumar, 2007) that influenced the work of Eychmüller and Domeisen (Chapter 7).

The reasons for using participatory action research to address particular issues vary (Waterman *et al.*, 2001). In a review of action research studies, Waterman *et al.* (2001) identify that such reasons include choosing an approach to research that involves and empowers stakeholders and participants; doing research with a practical focus on current problems; a synergy with the research process adopted with respect to theory generation; a cyclical process of feedback or the use of multiple methods; the educative aspect of action research; and, or, the recognition and attention paid to complex issues in complex situations. There is an active component to many of these reasons, reflecting the action element of participatory research. Such action leads to multi-level change (Ferlie and Shortell, 2001) for the individual, the team/group, organizational, and the wider system level. Individual interventions for change focus upon the individual health and social care practitioners delivering care. Team/group level change is concerned with the teams of individuals that provide the care for specific settings of groups of patients. More broadly, organizations provide the culture and climate within which change occurs. The wider system reflects the political economy and how this shapes care delivery within the region/country.

We use this typology to review the empirical studies presented in this book to look at where change has happened (see Table 16.1) and make some observations about the state of participatory research in palliative care and about specific challenges at specific levels.

Individuals

The large majority of the studies reported in this book do identify specific individuals with whom action and change has been directed. Even in the two studies where individuals have not been specifically identified as the focus of the research (Brazil, Chapter12; Heimerl and Wegleitner, Chapter 3), it is implicitly acknowledged that actions will need to be undertaken by individuals to effect the changes sought at broader organizational and community levels. The vast majority of research collaborators in these studies have been care staff, usually from a care rather than a medical background, such as nurses and care staff (also called personal care workers, personal care assistants, care assistants) working in long-term care settings. Volunteers and members of the public have been involved in studies (Eychmüller and Domeisen, Chapter 7; Froggatt, Chapter 14). Medical staff have been involved only within larger groups of care staff, rather than as lead collaborators.

The participants in these studies have generally not been the recipients of care. There were exceptions: family members were an active part of the study by Andrews

Table 16.1 Where is the change directed?

	Individual	Group/team	Organization	Wider environment/system
Developing end-of-life care with staff in two nursing homes (Hockley, Chapter 2)	Nursing home care staff	Staff teams (reflective de-briefing groups)	Nursing homes' processes of care	Included external primary care staff (to develop LCP)
Hospice and Palliative Care plan in Tyrol, Austria (Heimerl and Weigleitner, Chapter 3)			Inter and intra organizational working—hospital, home care, nursing homes	Regional stakeholders in funding and implementation
Community capacity development in long term care for Older People (Kelley and McKee; Chapter 4)	Long-term care setting staff; family members;	Palliative care team (created as part of research)	Long-term care organization	Hospice and other community agencies Alliance network
'Living with Dementia' project (Nicholson and Barnes, Chapter 6)	People with dementia, and family members	Created a group to collectively explore issues		Practitioners, managers, commissioners, third sector groups, and politicians.
Community palliative care in Switzerland (Eychmüller and Domeisen, Chapter 7)	Volunteers	Groups of volunteers created within project	Intra and inter- organizational work across agencies	Community networks of volunteers and statutory service working together
Addressing bereavement support involving people with intellectual disability (Read, Chapter 8)	People with intellectual disabilities; carers: nurses, parents, psychologists, doctors	Project focused groups	Advocacy organizations	
Palliative interventions and acute respiratory care (White and Lynch, Chapter 9)	Respiratory care nurses Palliative care nurses	Hospital respiratory care team hospital specialist palliative care team	Hospice primary care team Funding agency	

(Continued)

Table 16.1 (continued) Where is the change directed?

	Individual	Group/team	Organization	Wider environment/system
Improving pain management long-term care homes (Kaasalainen, Chapter 10)	Healthcare providers and managers	Care teams Resident council; Family council	Long-term care organizations	Regulatory and accrediting bodies
Working with staff and families in an aged care setting (Andrews et al., Chapter 11)	Care staff Family members	Care worker group Family group	Aged care organization	
Participatory action research with indigenous peoples (Brazil, Chapter 12)			Indigenous communities	Regional, provincial, and national partnerships
Gender and ethical perspectives in long-term care settings for older people (Reitinger and Lehner, Chapter 13)	Long-term care staff and managers	Inter-disciplinary team		
Peer education with older people (Froggatt, Chapter 14)	Older members of the general public; health and social care staff in public, private and voluntary organizations	Action group		
Hospital-based palliative respiratory care (Hynes, Chapter 15)	Respiratory nurses and palliative care nurses	Cooperative inquiry		

et al. (Chapter 11). Sue Read worked over a number of years with people with intellectual disabilities around bereavement (Chapter 8); older members of the general public have been active in public awareness work (Froggatt, Chapter 14); and people with dementia and their family members were involved in an appreciative inquiry study (Nicholson and Barnes, Chapter 6). However, with the exception of the appreciative inquiry work with people with dementia, the people involved in the studies were not actively living with a life-limiting illness or dying. This lack of active collaboration with patients/clients and users of services may reflect the characteristics of the palliative care population. As identified in other research approaches (Jordhoy *et al.*, 1999), issues of recruitment, attrition, and compliance shape the extent to which people with palliative care needs can participate in research. In qualitative interviews with older people in palliative care, Pleschberger and colleagues identified major challenges in including vulnerable people; for example how to access older people, the introduction of end-of-life issues in an interview, management of emotions, the presence of companions, and reciprocity (Pleschberger *et al.*, 2011).

Group/team

In all of these studies, attention was paid to the group/team as a focus for change. This either entailed researchers working with established groups of staff or creating new groups under the project remit. When working with established staff groups, a new form of space was often created as either there was the addition of a researcher to ongoing groups, or established groups used new times and foci to address the specific focus of the participatory research (see Hockley with the reflective de-briefing groups, Chapter 2; Kaasalainen, Chapter 10; and Andrews and colleagues from Tasmania, Chapter 11, for examples of this). The emphasis within palliative care on the team approach (Sepulveda *et al.*, 2002) may explain this level as a major focus in all the described studies.

Organization

Many of the studies reported in the book have focused on addressing palliative care provision in general care contexts that provide palliative care but without the specialist focus of organizations such as hospices. Many have been undertaken in long-term care settings in a number of countries (Australia—Andrews *et al.*, Chapter 11; Austria—Reitinger and Lehner, Chapter 13; United Kingdom—Hockley, Chapter 2; Canada—Kaasalainen, Chapter 10; and Kelley and McKee, Chapter 4). However, hospitals, too, have been the focus of the development of palliative care, such as in Ireland (Hynes; White and Lynch), working with specific populations of people requiring palliative care, such as people with chronic respiratory conditions. Some studies have explicitly sought to address change within and between organizations (Eychmüller and Domeisen, Chapter 7; Heimerl and Wegleitner, Chapter 3; Kaasalainen, Chapter 10; Kelley and McKee, Chapter 4).

Wider environment/system

Interestingly, the studies identified as addressing organizational change, explicitly, have also been the studies which have identified how to bring about social action across a wider system. The people who are involved in such change varies. The groups within the wider system that have been involved include healthcare staff external to the organization. From an organizational point of view they constitute the social environment, such as primary care doctors and nurses, hospice staff, statutory social care staff, strategic networks of care, funders at regional and national levels, regulatory and accrediting bodies, regional and national interest groups, and social and health-care political bodies.

Reviewing the studies using this typology makes it clear that the levels identified by Ferlie and Shortell (2001) are not used mutually exclusively in the research projects. On the contrary, it can be observed that, regardless of the focus of change in the study (be it about individual, group, organizational, or wider system change), it is apparent that all levels will ultimately be engaged with. The whole system is worked with reflecting the systemic thinking and practice that is so integral to action research (Flood, 2001).

Challenges using action research as an approach to social inquiry within palliative care

Throughout the chapters of this book a number of challenges have been identified when using participatory research within a palliative care context. We consider issues of relationship, initiating and sustaining participation, processes of change, the issue of power, ethical considerations, and engaging with sensitive topics.

Issues of relationship

Grant *et al.* (2008) consider that the majority of the challenges present in participatory research stem from the relational dynamic present within the approach. Action research is not a quick form of research. This is most likely because of its relational foundations and principles. It takes time to establish relationships and bring about sustainable change. Time is required to establish productive relationships between the researcher and the participants in their setting, regardless of whether or not the researcher belongs to the setting or is an outsider. Even if an 'insider' to the setting, relationships have to be re-established in light of new roles being undertaken within an action research study (Coghlan and Casey, 2001) (see Hynes, Chapter 15). The importance of working at relationships within an action research study cannot be emphasized strongly enough as, without conciliatory relationships, issues of power can be problematic (this is discussed in more detail later in this section).

Initiating and sustaining participation

Initiating and sustaining participation in participatory research studies in palliative care will be shaped by the people who are participating. As Casarett (2010) highlights, the decision making capacity within a palliative care population involved in research, particularly as people become frailer towards the end of life (Goodman *et al.*, in press), can cause challenges. Issues of competency may also be present, particularly for people with dementia, or fluctuating competency immediately prior to death. However, ways have been developed to address this and ensure that people with dementia are not excluded from participation (Dewing, 2007). The use of proxies is possible in some forms of research, but in terms of participation in action research they would not be appropriate. It is therefore not surprising that where people with palliative care needs have been involved it is much earlier in their illness, or post-bereavement (see Nicholson and Barnes, Chapter 6; Read, Chapter 8).

Individuals, whether staff or members of the public, engage in participatory research depending on their interest, available time, finances, and other commitments. There is the danger that participation becomes the 'new tyranny' (Cooke and Kothari, 2003), and in their enthusiasm the researcher misses practical constraints that shape the involvement by others. The benefits of the research may not be as obvious to participants as the burdens of participation. Partnership working is therefore important, as described in the chapter by Kelley and McKee (Chapter 4), and as they indicate, questions of empowerment of whom and by whom need addressing.

The extent to which subjects are able to volunteer for research participation is a concern to Casarett (2010); this can also be a challenge in participatory research when it is not always clear what is required. Even staff when agreeing to participate may not be aware how much time is required, and the extent to which changes to their own practice may need to be considered.

Traditionally, there is a large attrition rate when involving people with palliative care needs in research within a palliative care context, which is acknowledged to be challenging in itself (Casarett, 2010; Goodman et al., 2012; Jordhøy et al., 1999; Seymour et al., 2005; Steinhauser et al., 2006). The length of time involved with participatory action research studies is likely to mean that if people at the end of life are to be involved in participating it may need to be earlier in the disease process. Most participatory palliative care research does not directly involve people with advanced disease in the studies as active collaborators. Consequently, most issues of recruitment concern family and friends, and staff. However, one thing that a participatory action research study can achieve is bringing about a change in practice relatively quickly since change is designed to be part of the process. The emphasis on change is integral to the approach, and changes to contexts and situations will be made more immediately, thereby having the potential to make a difference to the participants themselves.

Processes of change

Bringing about change entails working with others in a setting. This can be a creative process that allows the identification of many practical actions in order to address the issue under consideration. However, conflicts will also happen and may be expected (Grant et al., 2008). As with all situations where change occurs there are differing responses to new ideas and actions.

Looking up the system, wider organizational responses to change may also be constraining. Where actions lead to a demand for resources that have not been anticipated, organizational management may be unprepared to support the outcomes of the research, leading to a stalling of the research and frustration on the part of the participants (Heimerl and Wegleitner, Chapter 3). Empowering people at the bottom of the hierarchy attributes power to them. When they make use of the power this may lead to conflicts within the hierarchy, a dynamic that needs to be discussed with leaders prior to commissioning an action research project.

Issues of power

Given such an emphasis upon relational dynamics in much participatory research, issues of power are ever present (Grant *at al.*, 2008). These can manifest themselves at any stage of a project, from initiation, design, planning, action, and review. These can be linked to the process of participation and change, or the insider/outsider roles occupied by researchers. As Andrews and colleagues describe in Chapter 11, the way in which power relations are enacted in a setting (in this case a long-term care setting for older people in Australia) can impact upon the research as well. By seeking to address the needs of family carers in this care setting, the involvement of this group of participants was initially shaped by the already existing dynamics between the care staff and the families. Only through separate collaborative working by the researcher with care staff and family members could a dialogue be developed to help a sensitization to the taken-for-granted dynamics.

Being an outsider in an action research study can also cause potential challenges to established dynamics of power. As described by Hockley (Chapter 2), and Reitinger and Lehner (Chapter 13), when working in an organization and providing feedback to the senior staff, it is easy to inadvertently challenge established hierarchies and threaten people's positions and status. Questions about who owns the research, as described by Brazil in his work with indigenous communities (Chapter 12), is yet a further articulation of the dynamics around power in participatory research that needs to be considered. Cultural competency and working with diversity is more explicit in some contexts than others (Brazil, Chapter 12; Kelley and McKee, Chapter 4), but attention to difference is important in any study. The OCAP model (Schnarch, 2004) referred to by Brazil (Chapter 12), offers a demanding challenge to researchers in other contexts, which warrants further attention.

Ethical considerations

Ethical considerations need to be addressed in all research involving human participants. Within palliative care a number of issues around ethical concerns have been described (Duke and Bennett, 2010). They identify that much attention has been paid to the protection of the rights, dignity, and safety of research participants in palliative care research but less to the needs of researchers and other staff. This observation is particularly apt within participatory research where, as we have identified, much research is undertaken with staff rather than patients or recipients of care.

Ethical considerations impact upon the organization when undertaking participatory research as well as individual participants. In some participatory studies the action or intervention is known at the start of the research and so all participants will be aware of what the focus of the work will entail. However, in other studies the action/s or intervention/s will only be known once the participants have started working together to identify the issues, and following that, the solutions. This has implications for formal processes of ethical approval. The lack of a predetermined intervention can be problematic for ethics committees who require specific information about interventions. It may be that a staged ethical approval will be required.

At the level of the organization and individual participating in participatory research, issues of informed consent need consideration. Risks to subjects involved in participatory research (Casarett, 2010) are more difficult to articulate as it is not always possible to identify what actions will be undertaken prior to the start of an action research study when individuals are invited to participate. If the actions that will be taken are not yet known then how can fully informed consent be given? As with the ethics committees it may be that a staged process offers an appropriate way to manage such difficulties, although process consent is another way round this, in which the participants can renegotiate the consent if an unanticipated event occurs (Streubert Speziale *et al.*, 2011: 449). Issues of anonymity and confidentiality also require attention. Particularly when working within organizations, there may be challenges to ensuring anonymity for participants, and where this cannot be guaranteed then this must be made explicit.

Inter-personal ethical issues are also present in participatory palliative care research—in the ethical space as described by Brazil (Chapter 12) and the relational ethics outlined by Kelley and McKee (Chapter 4). Organizationally, there can also be ethical issues around consent and information. Senior managers in an organization may agree to allow action research to occur in their organization, but may not be aware of the full implications regarding future demands for resources (as described by Heimerl and Wegleitner, Chapter 3).

Engaging with sensitive topics

A key issue raised about the challenges of doing palliative care research concerns the sensitivity of the substantive focus. This can result in concerns about the emotional aspects of doing research for the participants, supporting staff, and researchers (Duke and Bennett, 2010) (see also Reitinger and Lehner, Chapter 13). Even in an action research context an awareness of the potentially sensitive subject being addressed is required. However, this is not always a negative issue. Whilst recognizing the difficulty of ongoing emotional work particular encounters by staff with patients can be pivotal in creating momentum for change, as illustrated by Hynes in Chapter 15. It is therefore important that participants in action research studies in palliative care, be they people with life-limiting illnesses, bereaved family staff, or researchers, are provided with support, or access to it should it be required. This was outlined in the peer education study (see Froggatt, Chapter 14) where identified people were available, if required, to provide support for participations taking part in the workshops.

Responding to these challenges

The challenges outlined above that can be encountered in undertaking a participatory research within a palliative care focus or context are not insurmountable. They do, however, need to be addressed to ensure that the research is undertaken in as rigorous and high quality a way as possible. We propose two key principles to assist in addressing challenges, which will manifest themselves in study specific ways, and so need to be addressed appropriately to fit the context. These concern reflexivity and responsiveness.

Reflexivity

The importance of reflexivity has already been highlighted in a number of the chapters (Hynes in Chapter 5; White and Lynch in Chapter 9) and is inherent in participatory research. Kemmis (2001) and Marshall (1999; 2001) offer practical suggestions by which individual researchers can learn to pay attention to their presence and actions in, and on, the moment. This is related to the loops of learning identified by Hynes in Chapter 5. Whilst much reflexivity is done individually, there are ways to facilitate this within a group context through the principles of cooperative inquiry, as described by Hynes (Chapter 5). Assumptions about both palliative care and action research can be challenged by such an open-boundary inquiry. What these approaches offer is a way, either individually or collectively, to make visible what is often invisible with respect to gender issues, as described by Reitinger and Lehner (Chapter 13).

Responsiveness

The principle of responsiveness is closely related to reflexivity and integral to a participatory research approach. From the inception of a participatory research study through the process of carrying it out, there is a sense that responsiveness is key. The origin of any study like this needs to have a purpose and rationale based in 'practice' from an identified need. This is not research based on theoretical suppositions, rather it is undertaken to meet a need—a problem to be solved, a practice to be improved, or an intervention to be enhanced. In the process of doing participatory research, the willingness to build relationships, acknowledge and share power, and encourage participation are all vital steps in being responsive to the community with whom, and within which, the research is being undertaken (Grant *et al.*, 2008). Being responsive during the course of the research project requires changes in the plan where and whenever it seems appropriate.

In conclusion

This book has brought together an international perspective on the use of participatory research in palliative care. It argues the place of participatory action research within the critical theoretic paradigm and demonstrates the way in which such a research approach, increasingly taking its place alongside the more classical paradigms of healthcare research, can identify new knowledge about palliative care provision alongside practical actions that lead to sustainable change to support the care for people at the end of life. It is nonetheless a challenge for those excited by participatory action research when research achievements are measured within the positivist/quantitative paradigm. However, the studies reported in this book have shown how the integration of palliative care into other settings, such as long-term care settings and acute hospitals to a major extent, have succeeded as a result of using participatory action research as an approach to social inquiry. Wider system change has been described across regions of countries (Tirol, Switzerland) and in discrete communities and populations (indigenous communities, people with intellectual disabilities). This work has taken place in and across organizations and has implications upon individuals, be they (future) recipients or providers of care.

Building upon the lessons learned in this edited collection, we would encourage palliative care researchers and practitioners to seriously consider the relevance of participatory research to help find solutions for their concerns and issues. By describing the participatory research approach thoroughly from a methodological point of view, its rigour and quality, its challenges and its strengths, we do hope that this book will help to make participatory research better known and more widely accepted in the research community in palliative care.

Participatory research offers a practically focused, rigorous approach to addressing core issues of concern to practitioners and recipients of care. It is not easy and there are many challenges on the way, but it is rewarding. There are many areas and issues that still need to be addressed and we invite you to consider the relevance of what is offered here, to make a difference in your setting or area of concern.

Acknowledgements

We would like to thank the participants of the workshop about palliative care and action research held at the Collaborative Action Research Network (CARN) conference in Vienna, November 2011, for their lively discussion and challenging ideas, which have informed this chapter.

References

Casarett, D. (2010) Ethical Issues In Palliative Care Research. In: G. Hanks, N.I. Cherry, N.A. Christakis, M. Fallon, S. Kaasa, and R.K. Portenoy (eds), *Oxford Textbook of Palliative Medicine*, 4th edn, pp. 416–21. Oxford: Oxford University Press.

Chowns, G. (2008) 'No—You Don't Know How We Feel!' Collaborative Inquiry using Video with Children Facing the Life Threatening Illness of a Parent In: P. Reason and H. Bradbury (eds), *The Sage Handbook of Action Research*. 2nd edn, pp. 562–72. London: Sage Publications.

Coghlan, D. and Casey, M. (2001) Action Research from the Inside: Issues and Challenges in Doing Action Research in Your Own Hospital. *Journal of Advanced Nursing*, 35(5): 674–82.

Cooke, B. and Kothari, S. (2003) *Participation: The New Tyranny*. London: Zed Books.

Dewing, J. (2007) Participatory Research: A Method for Process Consent with Persons Who Have Dementia. *Dementia. The International Journal of Social Research and Practice*, 6(1), 11–25.

Duke, S. and Bennett, H. (2010) Review: A Narrative Review of the Published Ethical Debates in Palliative Care Research and an Assessment of Their Adequacy to Inform Research Governance. *Palliative Medicine*, 24(2): 111–26.

Ferlie, E. and Shortell, S. (2001) Improving the Quality of Health Care in the United Kingdom and the United States: A Framework for Change. *The Millbank Quarterly*, 79(2): 281–315.

Flood, R.L. (2001) The Relationship of 'Systems Thinking' to Action Research In: P. Reason and H. Bradbury (eds), *Handbook of Action Research: Participative Inquiry and Practice*, pp. 133–44. London: Sage Publications,

Goodman, C., Froggatt, K., and Mathie, E. (2012) End of Life Care Research Methods. *Methods Review*. London: NIHR School for Social Care Research.

Grant, J., Nelson, G., and Mitchell, T. (2008) Negotiating Challenges of Participatory Action Research: Relationships, Power, Participation, Change and Credibility. In: P. Reason and

H. Bradbury (eds), *The Sage Handbook of Action Research*, 2nd edn, pp. 589–601. London: Sage Publications.

Heimerl, K., Heller, A., Wegleitner, K., and Wenzel, C. (2012) Palliative Care und Organisationsethik: Partizipative Konzepte. In: R. Rosenbrock and, S. Hartung (eds), *Partizipation und Gesundheit*, pp. 408–17. Bern: Huber.

Hughes, I. (2008) Action Research in Healthcare. In: P. Reason and H. Bradbury (eds), *The Sage Handbook of Action Research*, 2nd edn, pp. 381–93. London: Sage Publications.

Kemmis, S. (2001) Exploring the Relevance of Critical Theory for Action Research: Emancipatory Action Research in the Footsteps of Jürgen Habermas. In: P. Reason and H. Bradbury (eds), *Handbook of Action Research: Participative Inquiry and Practice*, 91–102. London: Sage Publications.

Kumar, S. (2007) Kerala, India: A Regional Community-based Palliative Care Model. *Journal of Pain and Symptom Management*, **33**(5), 623–7.

Jordhøy, M.S., Kaasa, S., Fayers, P., Ovreness, T., Underland, G., and Ahlner-Elmqvist, M. (1999) Challenges in Palliative Care Research; Recruitment, Attrition and Compliance: Experience from a Randomized Controlled Trial. *Palliative Medicine*, **13**(4): 299–310.

Marshall, J. (1999) Living life as inquiry. *Systemic Practice and Action Research*, **12**(2): 155–71.

Marshall, J. (2001) Self-Reflective Inquiry Practices. In: P. Reason and H. Bradbury (eds), *Handbook of Action Research: Participative Inquiry and Practice*, pp. 433–39, London: Sage.

Pleschberger, S., Seymour, J., Payne, S., Deschepper, R., Onwuteaka-Philipsen, B., and Rurup, M. (2011) Interviews on End of Life Care with Older People: Reflections on Six European Studies, *Qualitative Health Research*, **21**(11): 1588–600.

Schnarch, B. (2004) Ownership, Control, Access, and Possession (OCAP) or Self-Determination Applied to Research: A Critical Analysis of Contemporary First Nations Research and Some Options for First Nations Communities. *Journal of Aboriginal Health*, January, **1**(1): 80–95.

Sepulveda, C., Marlin, A., Yoshida, T., and Ullrich, A. (2002) Palliative Care: The World Health Organisation's Global Perspective. *Journal of Pain and Symptom Management*, **24**(2), 91–6.

Seymour, J., Payne, S., Reid, D., Sargeant, A., Skilbeck, J., and Smith, P. (2005) Ethical and Methodological Issues in Palliative Care Studies. *Journal of Research in Nursing*, **10**(2): 169–88.

Steinhauser, K.E., Clipp, E.C., Hays, J.C., et al. (2006) Identifying, Recruiting, and Retaining Seriously-Ill Patients and their Caregivers in Longitudinal Research. *Palliative Medicine*, **20**: 745–54.

Streubert Speziale, H., Streubert, H.J., and Rinaldi Carpenter, D. (eds) (2011) *Qualitative Research in Nursing: Advancing the Humanistic Imperative*, 5th edn. Philadelphia: Lippincott, Williams and Wilkins.

Waterman, H., Tillen, D., Dickson, R., and de Koning, K. (2001) Action Research: A Systematic Review and Guidance for Assessment. *Health Technology Assessment*, **5**(23): 1–166.

Willke, H. (2005) *Systemtheorie II, Interventionstheorie: Grundzüge einer Theorie der Intervention in komplexe Systeme*, 4th edn. Stuttgart: UTB.

Index